MOVE TO IMPROVE

EXERCISE STRATEGIES FOR CIDP

By: Chris Willard

Move To Improve: Exercise Strategies for CIDP

Independently published in the United States of America

Dear fellow CIPD warriors and our loved ones,

This book is dedicated to those who have struggled with Chronic Inflammatory Demyelinating Polyneuropathy and to those who have supported us along this journey.

To the warriors, in the face of miserable circumstances, you have demonstrated amazing courage and tenacity, and your unflinching will to persevere is nothing short of inspiring. This book is a testament to your resilience and the hope you inspire in others going through similar challenges.

To our loved ones, your endless love and support are a testament to the power of compassion and empathy. During difficult times, you have been the rock that we needed, and your unwavering devotion has given us the strength to fight on.

This book is a testament to the bond that exists between CIPD warriors and our loved ones, a bond that transcends all of the challenges that this illness brings. May it give you knowledge, hope, and a sense of community.

With love,

Chris Willard

*CIDP is like the boss in an old-school video game —
the more you fight, the stronger it seems to get, so
spend your time & energy wisely*

LISTEN TO YOUR BODY!

TABLE OF CONTENTS

Introduction

An explanation of CIDP and the symptoms associated with it

Chronic Inflammatory Demyelinating Polyneuropathy (CIDP) is a rare autoimmune disorder affecting the peripheral nervous system, causing inflammation and damage to the myelin sheath surrounding and protecting nerve fibers. This damage results in a range of symptoms that typically develop slowly over time and may include progressive muscle weakness and atrophy, sensory disturbances such as numbness, tingling, and pain, and balance and coordination difficulties. In some cases, people who have CIDP may also experience involvement of their cranial nerves, which can result in symptoms such as facial weakness or double vision. In most cases, a diagnosis of CIDP is made after a thorough clinical evaluation, in addition to nerve conduction studies and other diagnostic procedures. The treatment may consist of a number of different procedures, such as immunosuppressive therapy, plasmapheresis, and intravenous immunoglobulin (IVIG) therapy. Early diagnosis and treatment of CIDP can lessen the severity of the condition's long-term effects and improve the overall quality of life for those who are afflicted.

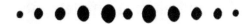

The importance of exercise for CIDP patients

Although it may seem counterintuitive to engage in physical activity when experiencing muscle weakness and other symptoms, regular exercise can help to improve strength, mobility, and overall well-being for individuals with CIDP. Exercise has been shown to have numerous benefits for individuals with CIDP, including increasing muscle strength, improving balance and coordination, reducing pain and inflammation, and enhancing overall cardiovascular health. Additionally, exercise can help counteract the negative effects of inactivity and prevent muscle atrophy, which can lead to further functional decline and complications.

It's important for individuals with CIDP to work with a healthcare provider or physical therapist to develop an exercise program that is safe and effective for their individual needs and abilities. This may include a combination of aerobic exercise, strength training, stretching exercises, balance exercises, and aquatic exercise. Modifications to the intensity, duration, and frequency of exercise may also be necessary based on the individual's symptoms and level of function.

Regular exercise can also help boost mood and reduce stress, which can be particularly beneficial for individuals with CIDP who may experience emotional challenges related to their diagnosis and symptoms. By incorporating exercise into their daily routine and establishing a consistent exercise regimen, individuals with CIDP can improve their quality of life and maintain their functional independence for longer periods of time.

In addition to being physically active, maintaining proper nutrition is essential for CIDP patients to support their overall health and manage their symptoms. Patients with CIDP can benefit from eating a diet high in protein, complex carbs, and healthy fats. They should also eat plenty of vitamin and mineral-rich foods, particularly vitamin B12, which can help mitigate nerve damage and inflammation. If you struggle to get the recommended amounts of vitamins and minerals in your diet, you can add natural supplements to your daily routine. Patients with CIDP may also benefit from avoiding processed meals, sweets, and unhealthy fats, all of which have been linked to increased inflammation. A registered dietician can work with you to create a tailor-made diet that promotes health and recovery.

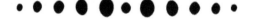

My journey

My journey with CIDP began when I was hospitalized for what appeared to be a stroke. I had all the physical signs of a stroke, but none of the normal markers were found in any of the subsequent tests. After a few months of treatment yielding only limited results, my neurologist theorized that I may be experiencing an autoimmune condition. After weeks of undergoing what seemed like every medical test possible, I was eventually diagnosed with chronic inflammatory demyelinating polyneuropathy (CIDP). With each symptom she ticked off the list, I recalled feeling each of the symptoms and began sinking deeper into a state of depression. Then I was given the devastating news that the best that can happen is for this to go into remission, but it could and most likely would return; there is no cure and no treatments that have been shown to be effective for everyone. I immediately thought of my family and how this would affect them the most. How would we pay the bills when I was the only one working? How was I going to play catch with my two little boys? How was I going to walk my daughter down the aisle at her wedding? How could I live out the dream that I shared with my young adult son of rebuilding a classic truck? Then I reminded myself that I'd been through worse, or so I thought.

An abbreviated personal history may be useful here. I was in a vehicle accident not long after I turned eighteen, and the impact compressed three of the vertebrae in my lower back. Even though I was warned that I might be bedridden, I was back on my feet and working in concrete construction within a year. This injury quickly became the reason behind every ache and pain that I felt over the next two decades. However, I now know that CIDP may have been the underlying cause for at least some of the suffering. At age 29, I was diagnosed with colon cancer, the very disease that had taken my dad when I was a child. Just over a year later, I was well on my way to full recovery when it was confirmed that I was in full remission. I could continue to fill a book with stories of the various illnesses that have plagued my body, but I'll write that one another day. I was a survivor. No matter what life threw at me, I was too strong to be defeated. But CIDP is different, and this mindset turned out to be my worst enemy. I ignored everything my body was trying to tell me, attempting to push through the pain, the weakness, and the numbness, ultimately defeating myself.

As I was experiencing one exceptionally debilitating CIDP flare-up I began researching alternative ways to manage CIDP. Through my research and while working with my medical team, I have found that functional exercise, nutritional adjustments, and emotional and mental awareness have been the most effective in managing my CIDP. Most importantly, I had to change my tendencies and learn to listen to my body. While it is important to keep moving forward, rest is just as important. If there are days when I don't feel like working around the house, exercising, or simply getting out of bed, I don't.

Understanding CIDP and Exercise

An explanation of how CIDP affects the body and muscles

In this chapter, we will explore how CIDP affects the body and muscles in more detail, as well as how physical activity can lessen its impact on daily life. The peripheral nervous system is responsible for transmitting signals between the brain and the rest of the body, allowing us to move our muscles, feel sensations, and control our bodily functions.

In CIDP, the body's immune system mistakenly targets the myelin sheath that surrounds and insulates nerve fibers, leading to inflammation and damage. This damage can disrupt the normal transmission of signals between the brain and the muscles, leading to muscle weakness and atrophy. This occurs when the muscle fibers are not being used as frequently due to decreased mobility and strength, leading to a decrease in muscle mass and size. Muscle atrophy can further exacerbate muscle weakness and functional impairments, creating a cycle of physical decline. The extent and severity of muscle weakness can vary depending on the location and degree of nerve damage. For example, if the nerves that control the muscles of the legs and feet are affected, an individual may experience difficulty walking, standing, or climbing stairs. If the nerves that control the muscles of the hands and arms are affected, an individual may have difficulty gripping objects or performing fine motor tasks.

In addition to muscle weakness, individuals with CIDP may also experience sensory disturbances such as numbness, tingling, and pain. This is because damage to the myelin sheath can disrupt the normal transmission of sensory signals from the body to the brain, leading to abnormal sensations or a loss of sensation altogether. Sensory disturbances may be particularly problematic in the feet and hands, where they can impact mobility and fine motor skills.

CIDP can also affect balance and coordination, as damage to the nerves that control these functions can lead to instability and falls. Individuals with CIDP

may have difficulty walking on uneven surfaces or changing directions quickly and may be at increased risk for injuries such as ankle sprains or fractures.
In severe cases, CIDP can also lead to complications such as respiratory failure or dysphagia (difficulty swallowing). This is because the nerves that control these functions may be affected, leading to difficulty breathing or swallowing.

It's important to note that the effects of CIDP on the body and muscles can vary widely between individuals and may change over time as the disease progresses. Some individuals may experience relatively mild symptoms that are easily managed with treatment, while others may experience more severe impairments that significantly impact their daily activities.
In terms of treatment, there are a variety of approaches that may be used to manage the symptoms of CIDP and slow disease progression. This may include immunosuppressive therapy to reduce inflammation and damage to the nerves, as well as physical therapy to improve strength, mobility, and balance. In some cases, individuals with CIDP may also undergo plasmapheresis or intravenous immunoglobulin therapy to remove or block harmful antibodies from the blood.

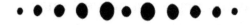

Patients with CIDP can greatly benefit from regular exercise

Regular exercise has been shown to have numerous benefits for individuals with CIDP. Exercise can help improve muscle strength, balance and coordination, flexibility, and overall physical functioning. Additionally, exercise may also help to reduce inflammation and oxidative stress, which are known to contribute to the progression of CIDP. In the following chapters, we will explore the benefits of exercise for CIDP patients in more detail.

Exercise can help to improve muscle strength and prevent muscle wasting by increasing the activation of motor units, which are groups of muscle fibers that are controlled by a single nerve cell. By activating more motor units during exercise, individuals with CIDP can increase their overall muscle strength, which can improve their ability to perform daily activities. Studies have shown that resistance training, which involves lifting weights or using resistance bands, can be particularly effective at improving muscle strength in individuals with CIDP. One study found that a 12-week resistance training program improved muscle strength and walking ability in individuals with CIDP, compared to a control group that did not engage in any exercise.

Exercise can help improve balance and coordination by increasing proprioception, which is the ability to sense the position and movement of the body. Balance and coordination exercises, such as standing on one leg or performing heel-to-toe walking, can be particularly effective at improving balance and reducing the risk of falling. In one study, individuals with CIDP who participated in a 6-week balance training program showed significant improvements in balance compared to a control group.

Exercise can help improve flexibility by increasing blood flow to the muscles and improving joint mobility. Stretching exercises, such as yoga or Pilates, can be particularly effective at improving flexibility in individuals with CIDP. These types of exercises involve holding static stretches for a period of time, which can help improve flexibility and reduce stiffness in the muscles and joints.

Inflammation and oxidative stress are thought to contribute to the progression of CIDP by causing further damage to the myelin sheath and nerve fibers. Exercise has been shown to reduce inflammation and oxidative stress by increasing antioxidant activity and reducing the levels of inflammatory markers in the blood. One study found that a 12-week exercise program reduced levels of the inflammatory marker C-reactive protein (CRP) in individuals with CIDP. Additionally, exercise has been shown to increase levels of antioxidants such as superoxide dismutase (SOD) and glutathione, which can help protect the nerve fibers from further damage.

Exercise is a valuable tool for individuals with CIDP to improve their physical and psychological well-being. It can help to improve muscle strength, balance, coordination, and flexibility, as well as reduce inflammation and oxidative stress, and improve overall physical functioning. By incorporating regular exercise into our treatment plan, we can improve our quality of life and maintain our independence. Exercise has been shown to improve mood and reduce symptoms of anxiety and depression. This is particularly important for individuals with CIDP, who may experience feelings of isolation and depression due to the impact of CIDP on their daily activities. It is important to work with a healthcare professional to develop an exercise program that is tailored to each individual's abilities and limitations, and to start slowly and gradually increase the intensity and duration of exercise over time.

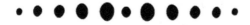

Potentially helpful forms of exercise for people with CIDP

Exercise is an important aspect of managing CIDP and can help improve physical function and reduce the impact of CIDP on daily activities. However, it is important to choose the right types of exercise that can be beneficial for CIDP patients. In a later chapter, we will delve deeper into the following examples of exercises that can be beneficial:

1. Aerobic exercise, also known as cardiovascular exercise, can be beneficial as it helps to improve cardiovascular health, promote weight loss, reduce inflammation, and improve overall physical functioning. Examples of aerobic exercise include walking, jogging, cycling, swimming, and dancing. It is recommended that CIDP patients engage in at least 30 minutes of moderate-intensity aerobic exercise, such as brisk walking or cycling, on most days of the week.

2. Resistance training, also known as strength training, can be beneficial as it helps to improve muscle strength and endurance, which can reduce the impact of CIDP on daily activities. Resistance training can also help reduce inflammation, improve overall physical functioning, and improve balance and coordination. Examples of resistance training exercises include weightlifting, resistance band exercises, and bodyweight exercises such as squats and lunges. It is important to

start with light weights or resistance and gradually increase the intensity and duration of resistance training over time. It is also important to note that you should be focused on functional strength training and not on becoming the next Mr. Olympia.

3. Balance exercises can be beneficial for CIDP patients as they help to improve balance and coordination, reduce the risk of falls, and improve overall physical functioning. Examples of balance exercises include standing on one foot, walking heel to toe, and standing on a wobble board or stability ball. It is important to start with simple balance exercises and gradually increase the difficulty and duration over time.

4. Flexibility exercises can be beneficial for CIDP patients as they help to improve their range of motion, reduce muscle stiffness and soreness, and improve overall physical functioning. Examples of flexibility exercises include stretching, yoga, and Pilates. It is important to start with gentle stretching exercises and gradually increase the duration and intensity of flexibility exercises over time.

5. Water exercises, also known as aquatic therapy, can be beneficial as they provide a low-impact form of exercise that can improve muscle strength and endurance, reduce inflammation, and improve overall physical functioning. Examples of water exercises include swimming, water aerobics, and water walking. It is important to always have someone present in case of emergencies when exercising in or near water and to work with a healthcare professional to develop a water exercise program that is tailored to the individual's abilities and limitations.

6. While exercise is a great way to improve physical health, it is important not to overlook the emotional and mental health benefits of exercise. Meditation and mindfulness, yoga, and creative expression are just a few examples that may be helpful for CIDP patients. In order to reap the benefits of emotional and mental health exercises, it is important to make them a regular part of your daily routine.

• • • • ● ●• ● ● • •

It is important not to overlook your emotional and mental health

Managing the physical and mental symptoms of CIDP is no easy task. Patients with CIDP often deal with physical symptoms like muscle weakness and exhaustion, but they may also have mental health issues, including worry and sadness. CIDP patients should exercise not only for the physical benefits it provides but also for the positive effects it has on their emotional and mental well-being.

Physical activity has been shown to improve mental health, and this is especially true for those with CIDP. Endorphins are substances produced by the body during exercise that improve mood and lessen the effects of stress and anxiety. Improved brain function and fewer depressive symptoms have both been linked to regular exercise. However, both factors can affect each other's health. The mental and emotional toll of dealing with a chronic condition like CIDP can have a significant impact on quality of life. Stress and anxiety can exacerbate physical symptoms for those with CIDP, but emphasizing emotional and mental health exercises can help alleviate both.

It's crucial to make emotional and mental health workouts a regular part of your daily routine if you want to reap the benefits. Here are some suggestions for making these workouts part of your routine:

If you're just getting started with practices like meditation or deep breathing for emotional and mental wellness, give yourself just a few minutes a day.

The best way to keep yourself motivated and aware of your success is to give yourself goals to work toward. You may try to meditate for ten minutes every day or devote an hour a week to yoga.

Consistency is essential when working on your mental and emotional well-being. You should try to practice at the same time every day, whether that's right when you wake up or right before you go to sleep.

· · ● ● ● · ● ● ● · ·

Embrace nature's healing power

The positive psychological effects of nature's power are real. Happiness can be yours in as little as thirty minutes a day; just remember to protect yourself with sunscreen and sunglasses. Sunlight has an intensity that is roughly 20 times that of typical indoor lighting. So instead of just staring out the window, enjoy nature up close and personal. You can even complete your workout outside; now that's a win, win. You could join fellow warriors in getting active outdoors while creating awareness and raising funds for research by participating in a <u>Walk and Roll</u> event near you.

Preparing for Exercise

Prior to starting any new exercise regimen, it is vital that you speak with your doctor

While exercise can be an important aspect of managing CIDP, it is crucial for patients to consult with their healthcare provider before beginning an exercise program. There are several reasons why it is important to consult with a healthcare provider before starting an exercise program for CIDP patients.

1. Safety: Consulting with a healthcare provider before beginning an exercise program is important to ensure that the exercises chosen are safe for you and your specific health condition. CIDP can cause muscle weakness and other complications, so it is important to choose exercises that are appropriate and safe for your level of strength and mobility.

2. Personalized exercise program: A healthcare provider can work with you to develop a personalized exercise program that is tailored to your specific needs, abilities, and limitations. This can help to ensure that the exercises chosen are appropriate and effective for managing CIDP.

3. Monitoring progress: A healthcare provider can monitor your progress over time and adjust the exercise program as needed to ensure that it remains effective and safe. This can help prevent injuries and ensure that you are making progress toward your health goals.

4. Medication interactions: Some medications used to treat CIDP may interact with certain types of exercise or physical activity. Consulting with a healthcare provider can help identify any potential medication interactions and ensure that your exercise program is safe and effective.

5. Addressing other health concerns: CIDP can be associated with other health conditions or complications, such as neuropathic pain, fatigue, or difficulty

breathing. Consulting with a healthcare provider before beginning an exercise program can help address any other health concerns and ensure that the exercise program is safe and effective for your overall health.

In addition to consulting with a healthcare provider before beginning an exercise program, it is important for you to listen to your body and make modifications as needed. Some exercises or activities may be too strenuous or cause discomfort or pain, so it is important to adjust the exercise program accordingly.

• • • • • • • • • • •

Guidelines for designing a safe and effective workout routine

Creating a safe and effective exercise plan is an important part of managing CIDP. It is important to choose exercises that are appropriate for the individual's level of strength and mobility and to make modifications as needed to ensure safety and effectiveness. Here are some tips for creating a safe and effective exercise plan for CIDP patients:

1. As discussed in the previous section, consulting with a healthcare provider before beginning an exercise program is important to ensure safety and effectiveness. A healthcare provider can help identify safe and effective exercises for managing CIDP and can work with the individual to develop a personalized exercise program that is tailored to their specific needs and abilities.

2. CIDP can cause muscle weakness and other complications, so it is important to choose exercises that are appropriate and safe for the individual's level of strength and mobility. Low-impact exercises such as walking, swimming, and cycling can be good options, as they are gentle on the joints and can be modified as needed. Resistance training exercises using light weights or resistance bands can also be effective for building strength and improving muscle function.

3. It is important to start slowly and gradually increase the intensity of the exercise program over time. This can help prevent injury and ensure that the

exercises remain safe and effective. Starting with low-impact exercises and gradually increasing the duration and intensity of the exercise program can help build strength and improve overall physical function.

4. It is important to listen to your body and make modifications as needed. Some exercises or activities may be too strenuous or cause discomfort or pain, so it is important to adjust the exercise program accordingly. If you experience pain or discomfort during exercise, stop the exercise and consult with a healthcare provider.

5. Incorporating a variety of exercises into the exercise program can help to prevent boredom and ensure that all muscle groups are being targeted. Incorporating exercises that target balance and coordination can also be helpful for improving overall physical function and reducing the risk of falling.

6. Staying hydrated is important for maintaining proper muscle function and preventing cramping or muscle weakness. Be sure to drink plenty of water before, during, and after exercise.

7. Warming up before exercise and cooling down after exercise can help prevent injury and ensure that the muscles are properly prepared for exercise. A warm-up can include gentle stretching or low-impact cardio exercises, while a cool-down can include gentle stretching or relaxation exercises.

Acknowledging and accommodating physical constraints

Understanding and working with physical limitations is an important part of managing CIDP. CIDP can cause muscle weakness, fatigue, and other physical limitations that can make daily activities and exercise more challenging. Here are some tips for understanding and working with physical limitations:

1. The first step in working with physical limitations is to identify them. This may include limitations related to mobility, strength, endurance, or balance. Identifying your limitations can help you tailor your exercise program and daily activities to your individual needs and abilities.

2. Once you have identified your limitations, it is important to develop strategies for working around them. This may include using assistive devices such as canes, walkers, or braces, or modifying your exercise program to accommodate your limitations. For example, if you have difficulty standing for long periods of time, you may choose to perform seated exercises or exercises that can be performed while lying down.

3. Setting realistic goals is an important part of managing physical limitations. This may include setting goals for exercise, daily activities, or other aspects of daily life. Setting realistic goals can help you stay motivated and make progress while avoiding frustration and disappointment.

4. Focusing on what you can do rather than what you cannot do can help you maintain a positive outlook and stay motivated. For example, if you have difficulty walking long distances, you may choose to focus on activities that do not require walking, such as swimming or cycling.

5. Listening to your body is important when working with physical limitations. This may include paying attention to signs of fatigue, pain, or discomfort and adjusting your activities or exercise program accordingly. It is important to avoid pushing yourself too hard or ignoring signs of physical stress or strain.

6. Seeking support and guidance from healthcare providers, physical therapists, or support groups can be helpful when working with physical limitations. These resources can provide guidance and support for managing physical limitations, developing strategies for working around limitations, and setting realistic goals.

You should ease into your workouts and build them up to your full potential. Some muscle stiffness or discomfort is to be expected while beginning an exercise program, but if the pain or discomfort persists or worsens, you should stop exercising and see a doctor.

Overcoming Obstacles to Physical Activity

Common challenges that CIDP patients may encounter when trying to exercise

Regular exercise is crucial for the management of CIDP. However, there are several barriers that CIDP patients may face when it comes to exercising. Identifying and understanding these barriers can help patients overcome them and stay motivated to exercise. In this section, we will discuss some common barriers that you may face when exercising and ways to overcome them.

CIDP patients often experience fatigue, which can make it difficult to exercise. However, regular exercise can actually help reduce fatigue and increase energy levels. To overcome fatigue, CIDP patients should start with low-intensity exercises and gradually increase the intensity and duration over time. They should also make sure to get enough rest and sleep and avoid overexertion.

Muscle weakness is a hallmark symptom of CIDP and can make it challenging to perform certain exercises. CIDP patients should work with a physical therapist to develop an exercise program that is tailored to their specific needs and abilities. They may need to use assistive devices, such as braces or crutches, to support their weak muscles.

CIDP patients may experience balance issues due to muscle weakness or sensory deficits. Exercises that improve balance, such as yoga and tai chi, can be beneficial for these patients. It is important to work with a physical therapist or a qualified instructor to ensure that these exercises are performed safely.

CIDP patients may experience pain in their muscles or joints, which can make exercise uncomfortable. However, regular exercise can actually help reduce pain and inflammation. CIDP patients should start with low-impact exercises, such as swimming or cycling, and gradually increase the intensity and duration over time. They should also listen to their bodies and avoid overexertion.

CIDP patients may have a fear of falling, especially if they have balance issues. This fear can make it difficult to engage in physical activity. CIDP patients should work with a physical therapist to improve their balance and coordination. They may also want to use assistive devices, such as canes or walkers, to support their mobility.

CIDP patients may feel discouraged or unmotivated to exercise due to their condition. It is important for these patients to stay motivated and engaged in physical activity to improve their health and quality of life. They should set realistic goals and celebrate their progress. They may also want to exercise with a friend or join a support group to stay motivated.

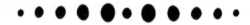

Strategies for overcoming these barriers, such as working with a physical therapist or using assistive devices

Strategies for overcoming barriers that CIDP patients may face when exercising are essential to ensuring that they can maintain an exercise program that is safe and effective. Some common barriers that CIDP patients may face when exercising include muscle weakness, fatigue, pain, balance problems, and mobility issues. However, there are several strategies that can help overcome these barriers and make exercising easier and more manageable for CIDP patients.

One of the most effective strategies for overcoming these barriers is working with a physical therapist. A physical therapist can assess the patient's physical abilities and develop an exercise plan that is tailored to their individual needs. They can also teach the patient proper techniques for exercising and provide guidance on how to progress their program as their strength and endurance improve.

Another strategy for overcoming barriers to exercise is to use assistive devices. This may include using a walker, cane, or wheelchair to help with mobility issues or balance problems. An exercise ball or resistance bands can also be used to provide support and stability during strength training exercises. These devices can help CIDP patients perform exercises safely and with less discomfort, making it easier to stick with an exercise program.

It is also important for CIDP patients to listen to their bodies and adjust their exercise program as needed. If they experience pain or fatigue during or after exercise, they may need to modify their program or take a break until they feel better. It is better to start slowly and gradually increase the intensity and duration of exercise over time than to push too hard and risk injury or exacerbating symptoms.

Other strategies for overcoming barriers to exercise include finding a supportive exercise partner or group, incorporating exercise into daily routines, setting realistic goals, and rewarding oneself for reaching milestones. By incorporating these strategies into their exercise program, CIDP patients can overcome common barriers and reap the benefits of regular exercise, including increased strength, flexibility, and cardiovascular health; improved mood and energy levels; and a better overall quality of life.

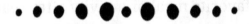

Suggestions for incorporating exercise into your daily routine

Making exercise a regular part of daily life can be a challenge for anyone, but it can be especially difficult for people with CIDP, who may face physical limitations and symptoms that make it harder to stay motivated. However, incorporating exercise into daily routines is important for maintaining physical function and improving overall health and well-being.

Scheduling exercise into your daily routine can help ensure that it becomes a regular part of your life. Patients should aim for at least 30 minutes of exercise per day and should try to do it at the same time every day if possible. This can help establish a routine and make exercise a habit.

Involving friends and family in exercise can make it more enjoyable and social. Patients can invite friends or family members to join them for a walk, swim, or other activity, or they can join a local exercise class or group. This can help provide support and motivation and make exercise more fun.

Using technology can help patients track their progress and stay motivated. Fitness trackers, apps, and other tools can help patients set goals, track their progress, and receive reminders to exercise. Patients can also use technology to connect with other patients or exercise groups and share tips and advice.

Being flexible is important when it comes to making exercise a regular part of daily life. Patients should be willing to modify their exercise routine as needed and be open to trying new activities. If you experience pain or discomfort during exercise, you should talk to your healthcare provider and modify your routine as necessary.

Rewarding oneself for reaching exercise goals can help provide motivation and make exercise more enjoyable. Patients can set up a reward system, such as treating themselves to a favorite meal or activity after reaching a certain goal. This can help reinforce the positive benefits of exercise and make it more enjoyable.

By incorporating these tips into their daily routine, CIDP patients can make exercise a regular part of their lives and enjoy the physical and emotional benefits that come with regular physical activity.

• • • ● ● • ● ● • • •

Motivation can be boosted by participating in activities that you enjoy

Finding the motivation to exercise regularly can be a challenge for anyone, but it can be even more difficult for individuals with CIDP, who may experience pain, fatigue, and weakness. One way to overcome this challenge is to find activities that are enjoyable and engaging. When you enjoy the exercise you do, it is more likely that you will stick with it and make it a regular part of your daily routine. In this section, we will discuss the importance of finding enjoyable activities to increase motivation and provide tips for finding activities that are right for you.

Participating in enjoyable activities can have a significant impact on motivation and adherence to an exercise program. When you enjoy what you are doing, it feels less like work and more like fun. This positive experience can lead to a sense of accomplishment and increased self-efficacy, which can then lead to greater adherence and improved outcomes. Additionally, engaging in enjoyable activities can improve your overall quality of life by reducing stress, increasing social connections, and promoting a sense of well-being.

Take some time to think about activities that you enjoy and find fulfilling. This could be anything from dancing to gardening to playing a musical instrument. Once you have a list of potential activities, try incorporating them into your exercise routine.

There are many different types of exercise to choose from, including swimming, cycling, yoga, and weightlifting. Experimenting with different types of exercise can help you find activities that you enjoy and that are appropriate for your fitness level and physical abilities.

Exercise can be a social activity, and involving others can make it more enjoyable. Consider joining a fitness class, a walking group, or a sports team. This can also provide accountability and support.

Setting goals can help increase motivation and provide a sense of accomplishment. When setting goals, make sure they are specific, measurable, attainable, relevant, and time-bound (SMART). Just remember to remain open-minded so that you don't become disheartened by setbacks.

Incorporate elements of fun into your exercise routine, such as listening to music, watching your favorite TV show or movie while exercising, or using fitness apps or games.

Celebrate your accomplishments and progress by rewarding yourself with something you enjoy. This can be as simple as taking a relaxing bath or enjoying a favorite snack.

• • • ● ● • ● ● • •

Establishing realistic objectives and monitoring our progress

Setting achievable goals and tracking progress is an essential part of any exercise program, especially for individuals with CIDP. Having clear goals and monitoring progress can help individuals stay motivated, build confidence, and improve their overall quality of life. This section will discuss the importance of setting achievable goals and tracking progress, as well as some strategies for doing so effectively.

Why Set Goals?
Setting achievable goals can provide several benefits for individuals with CIDP. Firstly, it can help them maintain focus and motivation throughout their exercise program. When individuals have clear, measurable goals to work towards, they are more likely to stay committed to their exercise routine. Secondly, setting goals can help individuals track their progress and celebrate their achievements, no matter how small. This can boost their confidence and self-esteem, which can have a positive impact on their overall well-being.

Types of Goals
Short-term goals: These are goals that can be achieved within a few days, weeks, or months. Short-term goals can be helpful for building momentum and creating a sense of accomplishment.

Long-term goals: These are goals that can take several months or years to achieve. Long-term goals can be helpful in providing a sense of purpose and direction and can help individuals stay motivated over a longer period of time.

Outcome goals: These are goals that are focused on the end result, such as losing a certain amount of weight or being able to walk a certain distance. Outcome goals can be helpful for providing a clear target to work towards.

Process goals: These are goals that are focused on the process of achieving a particular outcome, such as exercising for a certain amount of time each day. Process goals can be helpful for breaking down larger goals into smaller, more manageable steps.

Tips for Setting Achievable Goals
When setting goals, it's important to keep the following tips in mind:
Make them specific: Goals should be specific and measurable, so individuals can track their progress and stay motivated.

Make them realistic: Goals should be challenging but achievable. Unrealistic goals can lead to frustration and demotivation.

Don't make them time-bound: Goals generally should have a clear deadline or timeframe so individuals have a sense of urgency and can track their progress. However, CIDP patients never know when they may have a flare-up or relapse, and missing a deadline can be disheartening as a result.

Write them down: Writing down goals can help individuals clarify their objectives and stay focused.

Share them with others: Sharing goals with friends, family, or a healthcare provider can provide accountability and support.

Tracking Progress

Tracking progress is an important part of achieving goals. By monitoring progress, individuals can see how far they've come and make adjustments to their exercise program as needed. There are several ways to track progress, including:

1. Keeping a journal: Individuals can keep a journal to track their exercise routine, including the types of exercises they do, the duration and intensity of their workouts, and any progress or setbacks they experience. I have included a sample of My Daily CIDP Journal starting on page 62.

2. Using technology: Fitness trackers and mobile apps can be helpful for tracking progress and providing motivation.

3. Taking measurements: Individuals can take measurements, such as body weight, body fat percentage, or muscle strength, to track their progress over time.

4. Seeking feedback: Getting feedback from a healthcare provider, physical therapist, or personal trainer can provide valuable insight into progress and areas for improvement.

By setting achievable goals and tracking progress, individuals with CIDP can create an effective exercise plan that works for them. It is important to remember that progress may be slow, but every small step towards a goal is a success worth celebrating.

Targeted Workouts for People with CIDP

Exercising one's flexibility and range of motion through stretching

CIDP can cause stiffness and limited mobility, making it challenging to perform even simple tasks. Stretching can help improve flexibility, range of motion, and posture, as well as reduce the risk of falls and injury.

Before starting any stretching routine, it's important to consult with a healthcare provider or physical therapist. They can recommend specific stretches that are safe and effective for an individual's level of CIDP and physical ability. It's important to incorporate stretching exercises into an overall exercise routine but to also understand the importance of rest and recovery. It's important to remember to stretch gently and slowly, never pushing past the point of discomfort. Over-exertion can cause muscle damage and exacerbate CIDP symptoms, so it's crucial to listen to the body and take breaks when needed.

Keep in mind for the following examples that the 5 second hold time is only a recommendation; shorten or lengthen this time to fit your abilities. Getting down on the floor and back up again is a challenge for me at times, so I occasionally adjust by lying on my bed, a workout bench, or a sturdy table for the exercises that require lying. Do only the exercises that you're confident doing.

Arm Circles

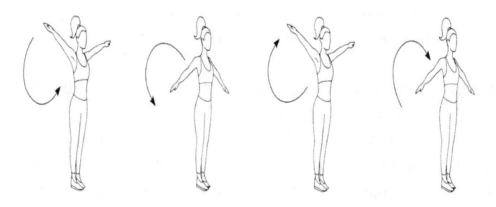

1. Keep your feet shoulder-width apart and your arms at your sides, parallel to the ground.

2. Start with modest, controlled movements of your arms in a forward circular motion, then work up to larger circles until you feel a stretch in your triceps.

3. After 5 seconds, switch the circles' directions.

4. Repeat until you feel that you've gotten a good stretch.

Cross Jacks

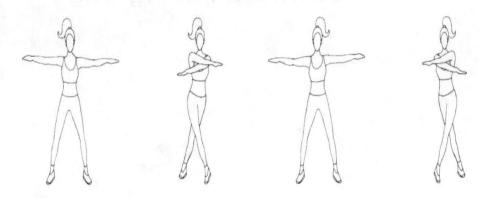

1. Stand straight with your feet shoulder-width apart and your arms up and extended out to the sides; keep your knees and elbows loose.

2. Step up and cross your left leg in front of the right, and your left arm on top of the right.

3. Hold for 5 seconds, then step again and return to the starting position.

4. Repeat, and reverse the position of your arms and legs.

5. Repeat until you feel that you've gotten a good stretch.

Downward Facing Dog

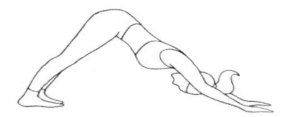

1. Get on your hands and knees. Your knees should be directly under your hips, and your hands should be under your shoulders.

2. As you exhale, straighten your legs to lift your hips into an upside-down V-shape. Your legs should be as straight as comfortably possible.

3. Press your hands into your mat and draw your shoulder blades inward as you take a deep breath. Your feet should be parallel and hip distance apart.

4. Relax your head to release the tension in your neck. Keep your neck and spine elongated and your shoulders broad.

5. Your legs should be as straight as possible, and your heels should be as close to the ground as possible.

6. Keep your spine straight, even if you need to bend your knees.

7. Hold for 5 seconds.

8. When you're ready to exit the pose, bend each knee to return to your hands and knees.

9. Repeat until you feel that you've gotten a good stretch.

Upward Dog

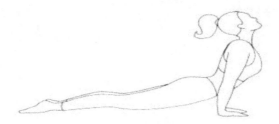

1. Lie in the prone position. Lie facedown on your stomach with your feet about a hip-width apart. Untuck your toes, and press the tops of your feet against the mat.

2. With your palms down, rest your hands alongside your abdomen, fingers pointing towards the top of the mat.

3. Lift your head and chest, lengthening your arms completely and press down through your palms. Lift the kneecaps off the floor.

4. Engage your inner thighs and calves as you lift your legs and pelvis off the mat.

5. Place your weight on your hands and the tops of your feet or toes. The rest of your body should be lifted off the floor.

6. Push your sternum forward and activate your arm muscles. Roll your shoulders back and down. Engage all of your arm muscles, bend your upper back, and fully activate your breath. Hold for 5 seconds.

7. Bend the elbows, release, and rest. Lower down slowly.

8. Repeat until you feel that you've gotten a good stretch.

Glute Bridge

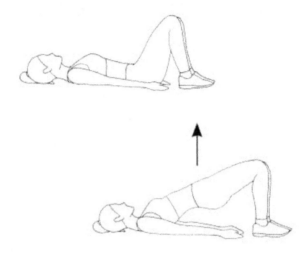

1. Lay down on your back with your knees bent and your feet flat on the ground. Your feet should be hip-width apart with your toes pointed straight ahead, and your heels should be about 6-8 inches away from your glutes. Place your arms by your sides with your palms turned up toward the ceiling.

2. Squeeze your glutes and your abs as you start to lift your hips toward the ceiling.

3. Raise your hips as high as you can go without arching your back. The goal is to raise your hips until your body is in a straight line from your knee to your hip and to your shoulder. Hold for 5 seconds.

5. Slowly lower the hips down to the floor.

6. Repeat until you feel that you've gotten a good stretch.

Hip Abductions

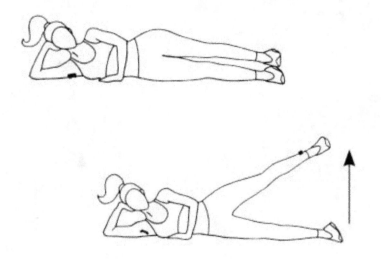

1. Lie down on your side with your legs stacked on top of one another and your toes pointed forward.

2. You can cushion your head on your bent left arm.

3. Gently raise your upper leg off of your lower leg without rotating your knee or spine.

4. Continue to raise your leg straight up until you feel strain in your lower back or oblique muscles. Hold for 5 seconds.

5. Return your leg to its starting position in a controlled manner.

6. Repeat until you feel that you've gotten a good stretch.

7. Switch sides and repeat.

Inner Thigh Leg Lifts

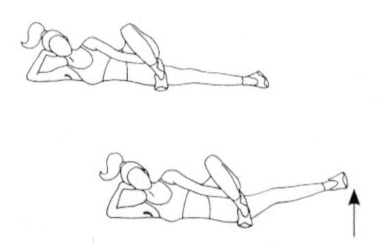

1. Lie on your side, lengthen your bottom leg, and cross your top leg over.

2. Flex your bottom toes toward your knee, lift the leg, hold for 5 seconds, and then lower it back down without letting it touch the floor.

3. Repeat until you feel that you've gotten a good stretch.

4. Switch sides and repeat.

Rotating Plank

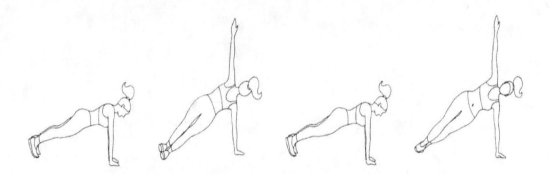

1. Place yourself in a plank position, hands on the ground beneath your shoulders. Straight body from head to toe.

2. Tighten your abs and glutes to hold up your body.

3. Reach your left elbow up toward the sky and slowly twist your upper body back, looking in the same direction.

4. Hold for 5 seconds, then return slowly.

5. Alternate sides until you feel that you've gotten a good stretch.

Fire Hydrants

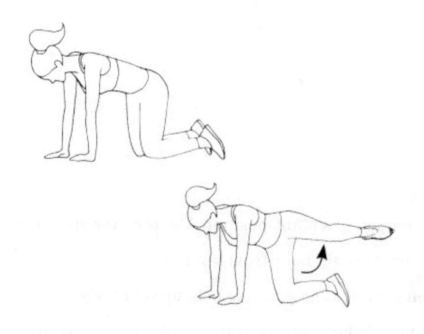

1. Get down on your hands and knees, with your wrists under your shoulders and your knees hip-width apart.

2. Keeping the knee bent, raise one leg up and out to the side until it's level with your hip.

3. Hold for 5 seconds.

4. Return to the starting position, and then switch legs.

5. Repeat until you feel that you've gotten a good stretch.

Strength training for muscle growth and maintenance

Strength-training exercises are an important component of an exercise program for individuals with CIDP. These exercises help to build and maintain muscle strength and endurance, which can improve overall physical function and quality of life.

When performing strength training exercises, it is important to prioritize safety. This may include starting with lighter weights, resistance bands, or no weights at all, using proper form and technique, and avoiding exercises that may exacerbate existing physical limitations or cause discomfort or pain. Additionally, it is important to work with a healthcare provider or physical therapist to develop a safe and effective exercise program tailored to your individual needs and limitations.

Functional exercises are movements that mimic daily activities and can help to improve overall physical function. These exercises can be particularly beneficial for individuals with CIDP, as they can help improve balance, coordination, and mobility. I have included some functional exercises that can be utilized with or without weights or resistance bands for additional strength building in the following pages. Keep in mind for the following examples that the 5-second hold time and 15 reps are only a recommendation; shorten or lengthen this time and number of reps to fit your abilities. Remember, only do exercises that you feel confident doing.

Boat Twists

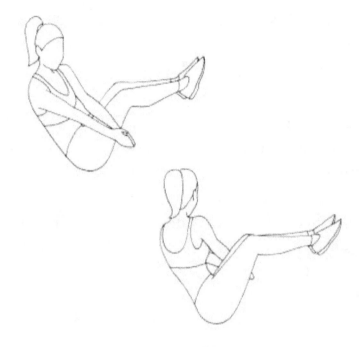

1. Sit down on a mat with your knees bent, extend your arms out to the sides, and lift your feet off the floor. You can rest your feet on a step or chair if needed.

2. Maintaining a slow and controlled motion. Twist your torso to the right and hold for 5 seconds, and then reverse the motion, twisting it to the left and holding for 5 seconds.

3. Repeat this movement until you've twisted in both directions 15 times.

4. You can hold a dumbbell weight or use wrist weights for added resistance if you feel comfortable doing so.

Push Ups

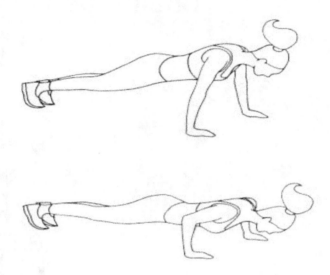

1. Begin with your chest and stomach flat on the floor. Your legs should be straight out behind you, and your palms should be at chest level with the arms bent out at a 45-degree angle.

2. Exhale as you push with your palms and heels, bringing your torso, chest, and thighs off the ground.

3. Hold for 5 seconds in the plank position—keep your core engaged.

4. Inhale as you slowly lower yourself back to your starting position.

5. Complete 15 reps.

6. You can wrap a resistance band around your shoulder blades, holding each end between your palms and the floor for additional resistance.

7. If a standard push-up is too challenging, try doing kneeling push-ups or wall push-ups.

Chair Dips

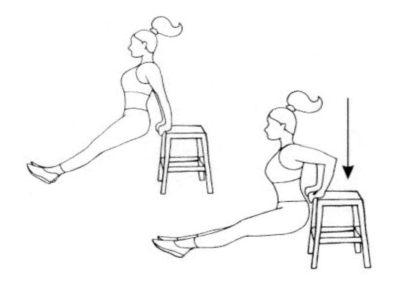

1. Place your hands behind you on a chair so that your fingers face forward.

2. Extend your legs and start bending your elbows.

3. Lower your body until your arms are at a 90-degree angle. Hold for 5 seconds.

4. Lift your body back up until your arms are straight. Hold for 5 seconds.

5. Complete 15 reps.

6. You can wear a weighted vest for additional resistance.

Dive Bombers

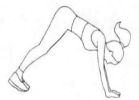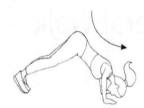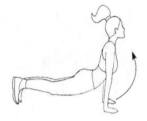

1. Begin with your hands and feet shoulder-width apart and your hips raised so that your body forms an inverted V.

2. Hold for 5 seconds.

3. Keeping your shoulder lowered and away from your ears, bring your chest forward between your hands as you bend your arms.

4. Continue to glide through as you straighten your arms and bring your chest up. Your hips will now be hovering just above the floor.

5. Hold for 5 seconds.

6. To finish the push-up, reverse the glide, raising your hips back up.

7. Repeat for 15 reps.

8. For added resistance, you can wear a weighted vest.

Lateral Walk

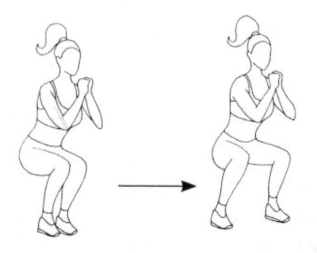

1. Stand with your feet hip-width apart.

2. Squat down into an athletic stance and take a small step to the left.

3. Keep taking small steps to the left, and then repeat on the right side. 4. Complete 15 reps in each direction.

5. For added resistance, wrap a resistance band around your legs at the ankles, knees, or both.

Lunges

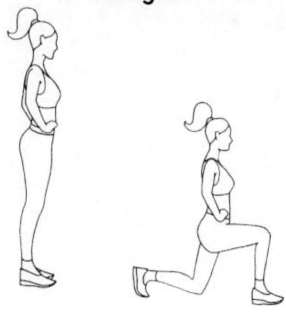

1. Stand tall with your feet hip distance apart, then take a large step backward with one foot. This is your starting position.

2. Hold for 5 seconds.

3. Lower the back knee to a 90-degree angle so both knees are bent, hold for 5 seconds, and then press up to the starting position and repeat.

4. Alternating legs, complete 15 reps with each leg.

5. For added resistance, you can wear a weighted vest or wrap a resistance band around your ankles.

Romanian Deadlifts

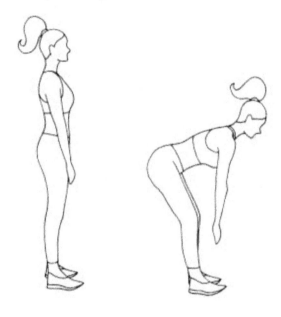

1. Stand up tall with your feet shoulder-width apart.

2. Hold for 5 seconds.

3. Push your hips back and lower your hands, while keeping your arms straight and your knees slightly bent.

4. Hold for 5 seconds.

5. Return to the starting position.

6. Complete 15 reps.

7. Hold two dumbbells or wear wrist weights for added resistance.

Single-Leg Pulses

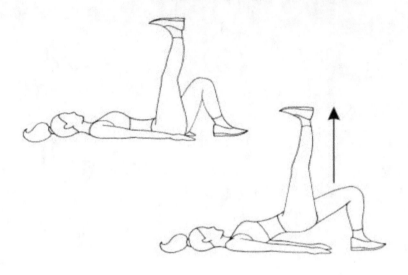

1. Lie on your back with your hands by your sides, knees bent, and feet flat on the floor (under your knees).

2. Lift one foot, extending the leg fully so it is roughly 90 degrees to the floor. This is the starting position.

3. Raise your hips, tightening your ab and buttock muscles to support the lift, until your shoulders and knees are in a straight line.

4. Hold for 5 seconds.

5. Lower your hips to the floor slowly and with control, keeping the leg extended, to return to the starting position.

6. Alternating legs, complete 15 reps with each leg.

7. For added resistance, you can wear ankle weights.

Squats

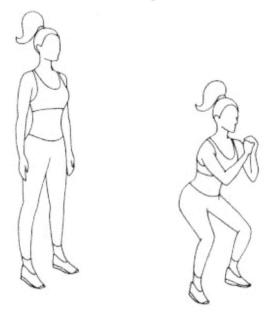

1. Start by standing with your feet shoulder-width apart, resting your arms down at your sides.

2. While bracing your core and keeping your chest up and your neck neutral, bend your knees and push your hips back as if you're going to sit in a chair. Your arms should raise up in front of you to be parallel to the floor.

3. When your thighs are parallel to the floor, hold for 5 seconds.

4. Then push up through your heels, back to your starting position.

5. Complete 15 reps.

6. You can hold dumbbells or wear wrist weights for added resistance.

7. You can place your back against a wall or place a chair under your buttocks if it helps you feel safer. Ideally, you don't sit down in the chair during this exercise, though.

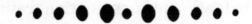

Cardiovascular exercises help to enhance heart and circulatory health

Cardiovascular exercise, also known as aerobic exercise, is an important component of any exercise program and can be particularly beneficial for CIDP patients. Cardiovascular exercise helps to improve heart health and circulation, increase endurance, and promote overall fitness. However, it is important to approach cardiovascular exercise with caution and to work with a healthcare provider to ensure that the exercises are safe and effective. There are a variety of different cardiovascular exercises that can be beneficial for CIDP patients.

Walking is a low-impact exercise that is easy to do and requires no special equipment. Walking can help improve cardiovascular health, increase endurance, and promote overall fitness. To make walking more challenging, you can try walking uphill or adding intervals of faster walking.

Cycling is another low-impact exercise that can be beneficial for CIDP patients. Cycling can help improve cardiovascular health, increase endurance, and promote overall fitness. If you have difficulty balancing on a traditional bicycle, consider using a stationary bike.

Swimming is a great option for CIDP patients because it is a low-impact exercise that provides resistance without putting too much strain on the muscles. Swimming can help improve cardiovascular health, increase endurance, and promote overall fitness. If you have difficulty with traditional swimming strokes, consider using a kickboard or other flotation device.

An elliptical machine is a low-impact exercise machine that simulates walking or running without impacting the joints. Elliptical machines can help improve cardiovascular health, increase endurance, and promote overall fitness.

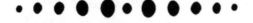

Reducing falls through balance and coordination training

People with CIDP should engage in balance exercises regularly because they can greatly benefit their balance, coordination, and posture. Stability and fall prevention can be achieved through training the abdominals, hips, lower back, and pelvic floor. Patients with CIDP can benefit from the following balance exercises:

Single-Leg Stability: One leg is kept bent and elevated slightly off the ground as the person stands on the other. Hold for 5 seconds. Alternate legs for 15 reps each. Close your eyes or try standing on a foam pad to increase the difficulty of the workout.

Walk on Your Toes: The heel of one foot should touch the toes of the other as the person walks in a straight line, as in the heel-to-toe walk. For added resistance, wear a weighted vest or hold dumbbells.

"Tree Pose" in Yoga: Standing on one leg while pressing the sole of the other foot against the inner thigh is the tree posture in yoga. The hands are clasped together in front of the body at shoulder height. Balance, posture, and focus can all get a boost from holding this position for 5 seconds. Wear ankle weights, wrist weights, or both for added resistance.

Sit-to-Stand: The goal of this routine is to get you to stand up from a chair without using your arms. Complete 15 reps. For added resistance, wear a weighted vest, hold dumbbells, or wear wrist weights.

Lateral Leg Raise: Lifting one leg out to the side while standing next to a wall or chair is a common workout. Hold for 5 seconds, then alternate legs for 15 reps each. Wear ankle weights for added resistance.

If you make these moves a regular part of your routine, you can boost your balance and stability and lower your chance of falling. Walking outdoors on varying terrain is a great, free way to challenge yourself and improve your mood.

However, it is crucial for CIDP patients to speak with a healthcare physician or physical therapist before commencing any fitness program.

Alternatively, you may try aquatic exercise

If a CIDP patient is searching for a low-impact way to improve their flexibility, range of motion, and overall physical fitness, aquatic exercises may be a good choice. Patients with CIDP can reap many rewards from participating in aquatic exercises, such as

Low-impact: Exercising in water is great for people with CIDP who may have trouble with high-impact activities like sprinting or leaping because of the low-impact setting it provides.

Less discomfort when exercising: CIDP patients may find it easier to exercise in water since their weight is dispersed more evenly throughout the water.

Water's resistance can aid in increasing flexibility and range of motion, which is especially helpful for people with CIDP who may feel muscle stiffness and tightness.

Aquatic exercise has been shown to increase heart rate and strengthen the heart and lungs, both of which contribute to better cardiovascular health.

Benefits for patients with CIDP include enhanced balance and coordination due to the unsteady environment of water.

Walking in the shallow end of a pool is a fantastic way to work on cardiovascular fitness, leg strength, and core stability.

For a low-impact cardio workout that's easy on the joints, try aqua-cycling, which involves riding a stationary bike in a pool.

However, there are some measures that should be taken to guarantee the safety and efficacy of aquatic exercise for CIDP patients:

To be sure that aquatic exercise is safe and appropriate for their unique needs, CIDP patients should check with their healthcare professional before beginning any new exercise program.

Wear necessary safety equipment; people with CIDP should always take precautions to stay safe.

Beginning with a low-intensity workout is recommended for CIDP patients, who can then work up to longer and more intense sessions as their strength and endurance improve.

Those with CIDP should keep an eye out for physical cues indicating weariness or pain in order to modify their exercise regimen accordingly.

To avoid becoming dehydrated, it is essential to drink enough water before, during, and after any aquatic exercise.

It is important not to overlook your emotional and mental health

By prioritizing emotional and mental health exercises, CIDP patients can not only improve their mood and overall quality of life but also reduce the impact of stress and anxiety on their physical symptoms. There are simple measures that you can take daily to protect your emotional and mental health.

Stress and anxiety can be effectively managed with meditation and other mindfulness activities. The goal of these methods is to help you relax and enjoy the moment by training your mind to stay in the here and now. Even if only for a few minutes a day, CIDP patients can benefit from making meditation and mindfulness activities part of their regimen.

Yoga is a nonaggressive practice that fuses physical activity, mental focus, and emotional calm. It can help you relax and unwind while enhancing your flexibility, balance, and strength. Yoga is a great form of exercise for people with CIDP since many of the positions can be modified to work around mobility issues.

Taking part in artistic pursuits like making music or writing can be a great way to lift your spirits and relieve tension. Writing in a journal, playing an instrument, or painting are just some of the creative options available to CIDP patients. In fact, this book itself is a direct result of my own free association writings. Various puzzles, such as the ones that follow, can also potentially help relieve emotional and mental stress.

The rules for sudoku are simple. A 16x16 grid must be filled in with numbers from 1 to 16, with no repeated numbers in each line, horizontally or vertically. To challenge you more, there are 4x4 squares marked out in the grid, and each of these squares can't have any repeat numbers either.

14				1		9	16			13		7	12		5
		11	1			5		6		7					
16	3	15				4			14					8	
			14		11	12	5		1						3
								11	13	2			15		
11								3	15					10	
		16		1	10	13					11				
		13			12	11		2				16			
3		7		5			11					8	14	4	
	1	2	15	16			6		12	8		5			
6	9		11	12	8		3	15		5		16	10		
5			8		11	2	14	16	7	3			15	9	
			9	2	4	15	10		5		14	8		11	6
15					12	5		8			6			13	
12	11	5			16	3	8		15	2		14		1	
8	7	6	2			14	1			10	11	4			15

Same rules except you're using numbers 1 to 9 to fill in the grid.

8		6						
	2	3						
9	4					3		2
	5			9			4	8
	9				5		3	
4	1		7			2		5
1		5		7	9	4	8	6
		9		1	8	7	5	3
7	8	4	6		3			1

Same rules except you're using numbers 1 to 4 to fill in the grid.

	3		4
	4	1	3
3			
4	2	3	

	3		1
4	1	3	

4		6			5			
				8				
2	8	1	3		9			
9					7	1		
3						2	8	
				5		6		
8			5	7				
		3			4			
1	7	9		2	6	3		4

				4				12							
		7		9	12					2					
1	12			7										16	
				10	6			8	15				14		
	5			8				4					7		
					2			9					6	15	
													16		
14		15		12	16		4				8		2	13	3
	16			6		13	3	14			1		8		12
									12		15				
	13		2				9					14	4	1	
			7					2							
12	3		16	15					2						
												11			
		4	10		9				7	5					
	2		1		6	12	11						15		

START AT THE TOP OPENING AND FIND YOUR WAY OUT AT THE BOTTOM OF EACH MAZE

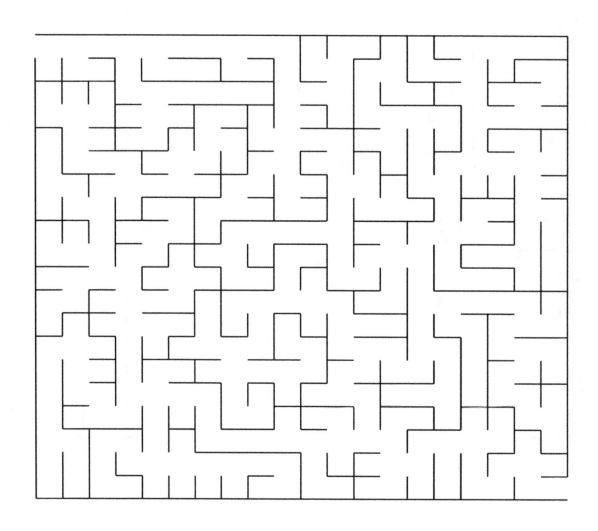

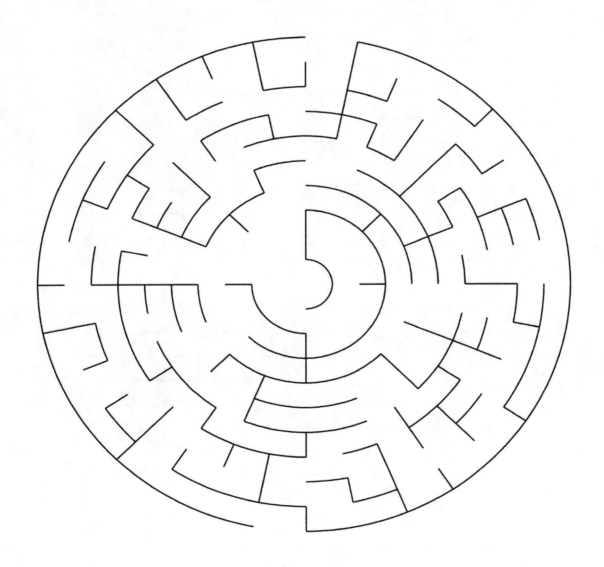

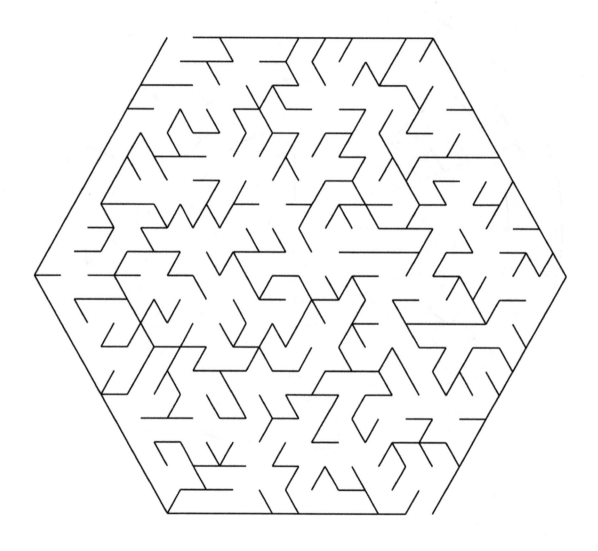

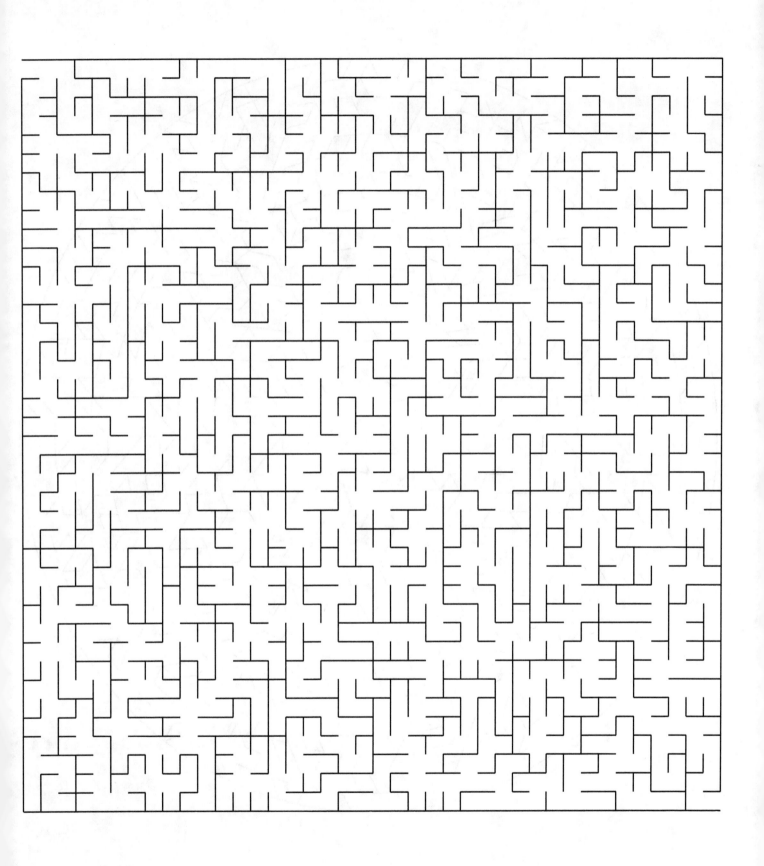

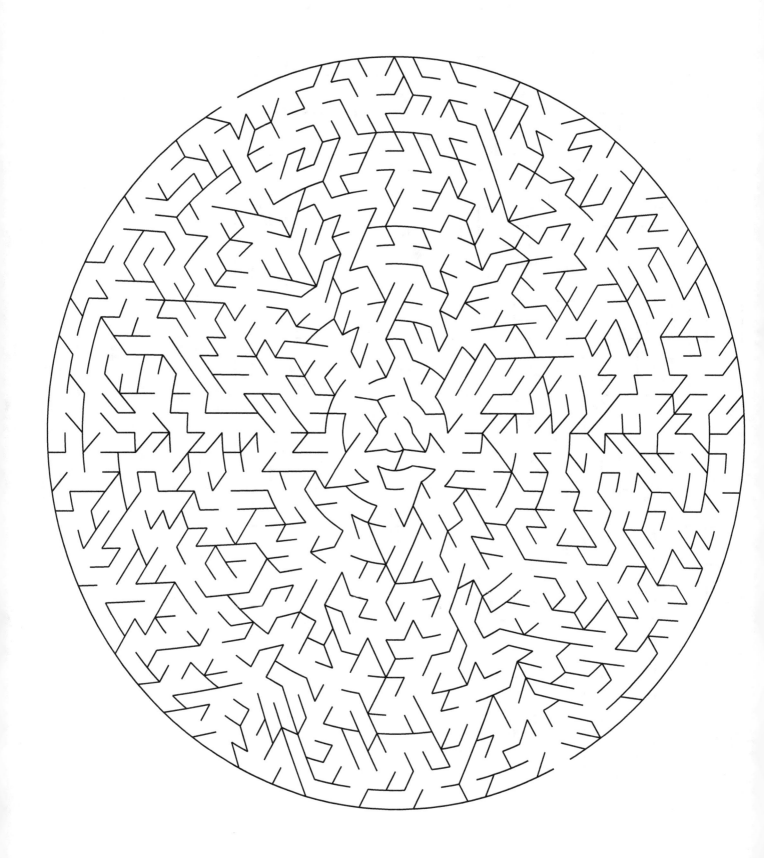

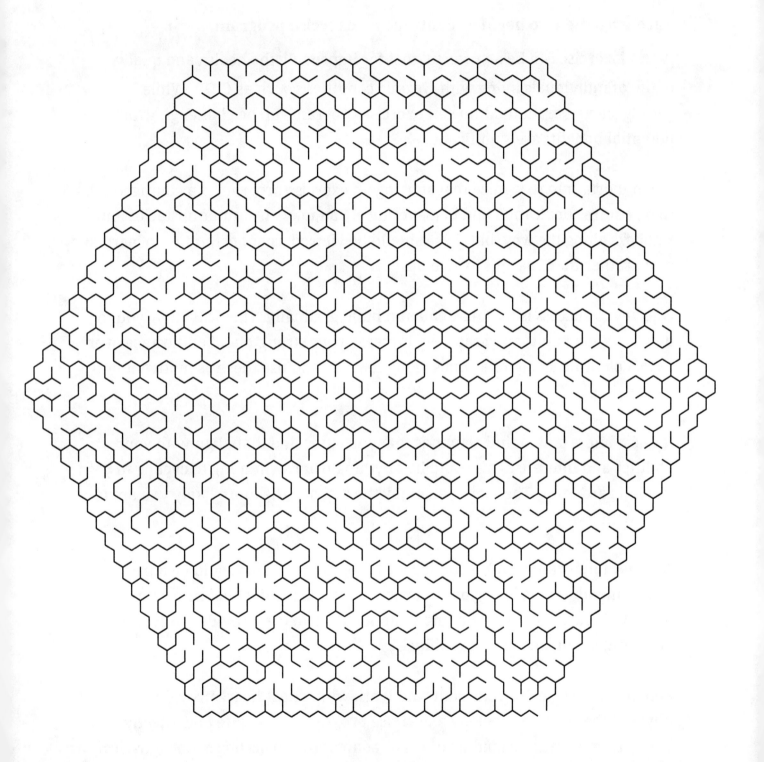

Final Thoughts

Encouragement to begin or continue an exercise program

Exercise can be a powerful tool for improving the health and quality of life of individuals living with chronic conditions such as CIDP. While getting started or maintaining an exercise program can be challenging, the potential benefits are significant.

It is important to recognize that starting an exercise program is a courageous step that requires dedication and perseverance. You may encounter obstacles and setbacks along the way, but these should be viewed as opportunities to learn and grow rather than reasons to give up.

One key to success is to start small and build gradually. This will allow you to develop good habits and gradually increase your strength and endurance over time. Celebrate small milestones along the way and use these as motivation to keep going.

It's also important to find activities that you enjoy and that align with your abilities and interests. This could be anything from swimming to cycling to yoga to even gardening. The more you enjoy the activity, the more likely you are to stick with it.

Another important factor is finding a support system. This could be a friend or family member who joins you for exercise sessions, or it could be a support group for individuals with CIDP. Having a support system can provide motivation, encouragement, and accountability.

Remember to listen to your body and work with a healthcare provider or physical therapist to develop an exercise program that is safe and effective for you. This may include modifications or adaptations to accommodate physical limitations.

Finally, it's important to be patient with yourself and celebrate your progress, no matter how small. Exercise is a journey, not a destination, and every step forward is a step in the right direction. Stay committed, stay positive, and keep moving forward. With time and dedication, the benefits of exercise for CIDP patients can be life-changing.

• • • ● ● • ● ● • •

Where to find more information and help

There are several resources available for further information and support for CIDP patients who are interested in starting an exercise program.

Here are a few:

1. Charcot-Marie-Tooth Association (CMTA) - The CMTA is a nonprofit organization that provides information and support to individuals with CIDP and related disorders. Their website, cmtausa.org includes a section on exercise and physical therapy for CMT/CIDP patients.

2. Muscular Dystrophy Association (MDA) - The MDA is a nonprofit organization that provides support and resources to individuals with neuromuscular disorders. Their website, mda.org includes a section on physical therapy and exercise for individuals with neuromuscular diseases.

3. National Institute of Neurological Disorders and Stroke (NINDS) - The NINDS is a government organization that conducts and supports research on neurological disorders. Their website, ninds.nih.gov includes information on CIDP and related disorders, including treatment and management options.

4. Physical therapy clinics - Physical therapy clinics are a great resource for CIDP patients who are interested in starting an exercise program. A physical therapist can assess the patient's individual needs and develop a personalized exercise plan to improve strength, flexibility, and balance.

5. Support groups - Support groups can provide valuable emotional support and advice for individuals with CIDP who are interested in starting an exercise program. The CMTA and MDA both offer support groups for individuals with

neuromuscular disorders. Various social media support groups of fellow patients, such as CIDPSupport and the official GBS/CIDP Foundation Facebook page, are also great resources.

6. Online resources - There are several online resources available for CIDP patients who are interested in starting an exercise program, including YouTube videos and online exercise classes. However, it is important to consult with a healthcare provider before starting any new exercise program, even if it is online.

7. The GBS-CIDP Foundation International is a non-profit organization dedicated to supporting patients and families affected by Guillain-Barré syndrome (GBS), chronic inflammatory demyelinating polyneuropathy (CIDP), and related syndromes through research, education, advocacy, and patient services. The website, gbs-cidp.org provides information about these conditions, including their symptoms, causes, and treatment options, as well as resources for patients, caregivers, and healthcare professionals. The site also hosts a community forum where individuals affected by GBS, CIDP, and related conditions can connect and share their experiences.

I would love to connect with you on Instagram.

CHRISWILLARDAUTHOR

Record Your CIDP Journey

Keeping track of your symptoms and progress is simplified with a journal. I have included a sample of My Daily CIDP Journal in the pages that follow.

My Daily CIDP Journal can be purchased separately at Amazon, Barnes & Noble, and many other book retailers. If you can't find it locally, ask a manager to order it. You can also request a free printable PDF by emailing me at cwillardauthor@gmail.com .

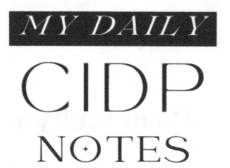

MY DAILY
CIDP
NOTES

_____
_____
_____
_____
_____
_____
_____
_____
_____
_____
_____
_____
_____
_____
_____
_____
_____
_____
_____
_____

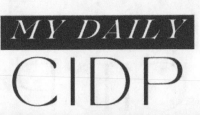

CIDP

MY GOALS	MY MOTIVATION

START	MY ACTION PLAN	FINISH

MY ULTIMATE REWARD

MY DAILY
CIDP

TODAY IS _____

WOKE UP FEELING

☺ ☺ ☺ ☺ ☺

I SLEPT (HOURS)
_____

I WOKE UP AT
_____

GOING TO BED FEELING

☺ ☺ ☺ ☺ ☺

I WAS ACTIVE (HOURS)
_____

I AM GOING TO BED AT
_____

TODAY I WOULD LIKE TO

01 _____

02 _____

03 _____

GOAL ACCOMPLISHED?

_____

_____

_____

SYMPTOMS THIS MORNING

_____
_____
_____
_____
_____
_____
_____
_____
_____

SYMPTOMS THIS EVENING

_____
_____
_____
_____
_____
_____
_____
_____
_____

WATER ⬡⬡⬡⬡⬡⬡⬡⬡⬡

MEALS 🍽 🍽 🍽 🍽 🍽

MY DAILY

CIDP

BEFORE WORKOUT

TARGET WORKOUT LENGTH: _____

AFTER WORKOUT

ACTUAL WORKOUT LENGTH: _____

EXERCISE	SETS	REPS	RESISTANCE AMOUNT & TYPE

MEAL		PORTION	TIME
BREAKFAST			
SNACK			
LUNCH			
SNACK			
DINNER			

NOTES:

_____

_____

_____

_____

MY DAILY
CIDP

TODAY IS _____

WOKE UP FEELING

☺ ☺ ☺ ☺ ☺

I SLEPT (HOURS) _____

I WOKE UP AT _____

GOING TO BED FEELING

☺ ☺ ☺ ☺ ☺

I WAS ACTIVE (HOURS) _____

I AM GOING TO BED AT _____

TODAY I WOULD LIKE TO

GOAL ACCOMPLISHED?

01 _____

02 _____

03 _____

SYMPTOMS THIS MORNING

_____
_____
_____
_____
_____
_____
_____
_____
_____

SYMPTOMS THIS EVENING

_____
_____
_____
_____
_____
_____
_____
_____
_____

WATER ○○○○○○○○○

MEALS 🍽 🍽 🍽 🍽 🍽

MY DAILY
CIDP

BEFORE WORKOUT

AFTER WORKOUT

TARGET WORKOUT LENGTH: _____

ACTUAL WORKOUT LENGTH: _____

EXERCISE	SETS	REPS	RESISTANCE AMOUNT & TYPE

MEAL		PORTION	TIME
BREAKFAST			
SNACK			
LUNCH			
SNACK			
DINNER			

NOTES:

_____

_____

_____

_____

MY DAILY
CIDP

TODAY IS _____

WOKE UP FEELING

☺ ☺ ☺ ☺ ☺

I SLEPT (HOURS)
_____

I WOKE UP AT
_____

GOING TO BED FEELING

☺ ☺ ☺ ☺ ☺

I WAS ACTIVE (HOURS)
_____

I AM GOING TO BED AT
_____

TODAY I WOULD LIKE TO

GOAL ACCOMPLISHED?
_____

01 _____

02 _____

03 _____

SYMPTOMS THIS MORNING

_____

_____

_____

_____

_____

_____

_____

_____

_____

SYMPTOMS THIS EVENING

_____

_____

_____

_____

_____

_____

_____

_____

_____

WATER ◊ ◊ ◊ ◊ ◊ ◊ ◊ ◊   MEALS 🍽 🍽 🍽 🍽 🍽

MY DAILY
CIDP

BEFORE WORKOUT

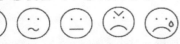

AFTER WORKOUT

TARGET WORKOUT LENGTH: _____

ACTUAL WORKOUT LENGTH: _____

EXERCISE	SETS	REPS	RESISTANCE AMOUNT & TYPE

MEAL		PORTION	TIME
BREAKFAST			
SNACK			
LUNCH			
SNACK			
DINNER			

NOTES:

_____

_____

_____

_____

MY DAILY
CIDP

TODAY IS _____

WOKE UP FEELING

😊 🙂 😐 😠 😢

I SLEPT (HOURS)
_____

I WOKE UP AT
_____

GOING TO BED FEELING

😊 🙂 😐 😠 😢

I WAS ACTIVE (HOURS)
_____

I AM GOING TO BED AT
_____

TODAY I WOULD LIKE TO

01 _____

02 _____

03 _____

GOAL ACCOMPLISHED?

_____

SYMPTOMS THIS MORNING

_____
_____
_____
_____
_____
_____
_____
_____
_____

SYMPTOMS THIS EVENING

_____
_____
_____
_____
_____
_____
_____
_____
_____

WATER ⬦⬦⬦⬦⬦⬦⬦⬦⬦

MEALS 🍽️🍽️🍽️🍽️🍽️

MY DAILY

CIDP

BEFORE WORKOUT

AFTER WORKOUT

TARGET WORKOUT LENGTH: _____

ACTUAL WORKOUT LENGTH: _____

EXERCISE	SETS	REPS	RESISTANCE AMOUNT & TYPE

MEAL		PORTION	TIME
BREAKFAST			
SNACK			
LUNCH			
SNACK			
DINNER			

NOTES:

_____

_____

_____

_____

MY DAILY
CIDP

TODAY IS _____

WOKE UP FEELING

☺ ☺ ☺ ☹ ☹

I SLEPT (HOURS)
_____

I WOKE UP AT
_____

GOING TO BED FEELING

☺ ☺ ☺ ☹ ☹

I WAS ACTIVE (HOURS)
_____

I AM GOING TO BED AT
_____

TODAY I WOULD LIKE TO

01 _____

02 _____

03 _____

GOAL ACCOMPLISHED?

_____

_____

_____

_____

SYMPTOMS THIS MORNING

_____

_____

_____

_____

_____

_____

_____

_____

_____

SYMPTOMS THIS EVENING

_____

_____

_____

_____

_____

_____

_____

_____

_____

WATER ○○○○○○○○○

MEALS 🍽 🍽 🍽 🍽 🍽

MY DAILY
CIDP

BEFORE WORKOUT

TARGET WORKOUT LENGTH: _____

AFTER WORKOUT

ACTUAL WORKOUT LENGTH: _____

EXERCISE	SETS	REPS	RESISTANCE AMOUNT & TYPE

MEAL		PORTION	TIME
BREAKFAST			
SNACK			
LUNCH			
SNACK			
DINNER			

NOTES:

_____

_____

_____

_____

MY DAILY
CIDP

TODAY IS _____

WOKE UP FEELING
☺ 🙂 😐 😠 😢

I SLEPT (HOURS) _____

I WOKE UP AT _____

GOING TO BED FEELING
☺ 🙂 😐 😠 😢

I WAS ACTIVE (HOURS) _____

I AM GOING TO BED AT _____

TODAY I WOULD LIKE TO

GOAL ACCOMPLISHED?

01 _____

02 _____

03 _____

SYMPTOMS THIS MORNING

_____
_____
_____
_____
_____
_____
_____
_____

SYMPTOMS THIS EVENING

_____
_____
_____
_____
_____
_____
_____
_____

WATER 💧💧💧💧💧💧💧💧

MEALS 🍽🍽🍽🍽🍽

BEFORE WORKOUT

AFTER WORKOUT

TARGET WORKOUT LENGTH: _____

ACTUAL WORKOUT LENGTH: _____

EXERCISE	SETS	REPS	RESISTANCE AMOUNT & TYPE

MEAL		PORTION	TIME
BREAKFAST			
SNACK			
LUNCH			
SNACK			
DINNER			

NOTES:

_____

_____

_____

_____

CIDP

TODAY IS _____

WOKE UP FEELING

☺ ☺ ☺ ☹ ☹

I SLEPT (HOURS)
_____

I WOKE UP AT
_____

GOING TO BED FEELING

☺ ☺ ☺ ☹ ☹

I WAS ACTIVE (HOURS)
_____

I AM GOING TO BED AT
_____

TODAY I WOULD LIKE TO

01 _____

02 _____

03 _____

GOAL ACCOMPLISHED?

SYMPTOMS THIS MORNING

_____
_____
_____
_____
_____
_____
_____
_____
_____

SYMPTOMS THIS EVENING

_____
_____
_____
_____
_____
_____
_____
_____
_____

WATER ○○○○○○○○○

MEALS 🍽 🍽 🍽 🍽 🍽

MY DAILY

CIDP

BEFORE WORKOUT

AFTER WORKOUT

TARGET WORKOUT LENGTH: _____

ACTUAL WORKOUT LENGTH: _____

EXERCISE	SETS	REPS	RESISTANCE AMOUNT & TYPE

MEAL		PORTION	TIME
BREAKFAST			
SNACK			
LUNCH			
SNACK			
DINNER			

NOTES:

_____

_____

_____

_____

CIDP

TODAY IS _____

WOKE UP FEELING

😊 🙂 😐 😠 😢

I SLEPT (HOURS) _____

I WOKE UP AT _____

GOING TO BED FEELING

😊 🙂 😐 😠 😢

I WAS ACTIVE (HOURS) _____

I AM GOING TO BED AT _____

TODAY I WOULD LIKE TO

01 _____

02 _____

03 _____

GOAL ACCOMPLISHED?

SYMPTOMS THIS MORNING

_____
_____
_____
_____
_____
_____
_____
_____
_____

SYMPTOMS THIS EVENING

_____
_____
_____
_____
_____
_____
_____
_____
_____

WATER ⬡⬡⬡⬡⬡⬡⬡⬡

MEALS 🍽️ 🍽️ 🍽️ 🍽️ 🍽️

BEFORE WORKOUT

   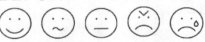

AFTER WORKOUT

TARGET WORKOUT LENGTH: _____   ACTUAL WORKOUT LENGTH: _____

EXERCISE	SETS	REPS	RESISTANCE AMOUNT & TYPE

MEAL		PORTION	TIME
BREAKFAST			
SNACK			
LUNCH			
SNACK			
DINNER			

NOTES:

_____

_____

_____

_____

MY DAILY
CIDP

TODAY IS _____

WOKE UP FEELING

☺ 😕 😐 😣 😢

I SLEPT (HOURS)
_____

I WOKE UP AT
_____

GOING TO BED FEELING

☺ 😕 😐 😣 😢

I WAS ACTIVE (HOURS)
_____

I AM GOING TO BED AT
_____

TODAY I WOULD LIKE TO

01 _____

02 _____

03 _____

GOAL ACCOMPLISHED?

SYMPTOMS THIS MORNING

_____
_____
_____
_____
_____
_____
_____
_____
_____

SYMPTOMS THIS EVENING

_____
_____
_____
_____
_____
_____
_____
_____
_____

WATER ⬭⬭⬭⬭⬭⬭⬭⬭   MEALS 🍽️🍽️🍽️🍽️🍽️

MY DAILY

CIDP

BEFORE WORKOUT

AFTER WORKOUT

TARGET WORKOUT LENGTH: _____

ACTUAL WORKOUT LENGTH: _____

EXERCISE	SETS	REPS	RESISTANCE AMOUNT & TYPE

MEAL		PORTION	TIME
BREAKFAST			
SNACK			
LUNCH			
SNACK			
DINNER			

NOTES:

_____

_____

_____

_____

MY DAILY
CIDP

TODAY IS _____

WOKE UP FEELING

☺ ☺ ☺ ☹ ☹

I SLEPT (HOURS) _____

I WOKE UP AT _____

GOING TO BED FEELING

☺ ☺ ☺ ☹ ☹

I WAS ACTIVE (HOURS) _____

I AM GOING TO BED AT _____

TODAY I WOULD LIKE TO

GOAL ACCOMPLISHED?

01 _____

02 _____

03 _____

SYMPTOMS THIS MORNING

_____
_____
_____
_____
_____
_____
_____
_____
_____

SYMPTOMS THIS EVENING

_____
_____
_____
_____
_____
_____
_____
_____
_____

WATER ○○○○○○○○

MEALS 🍽 🍽 🍽 🍽 🍽

MY DAILY
CIDP

BEFORE WORKOUT

AFTER WORKOUT

TARGET WORKOUT LENGTH: _____

ACTUAL WORKOUT LENGTH: _____

EXERCISE	SETS	REPS	RESISTANCE AMOUNT & TYPE

MEAL		PORTION	TIME
BREAKFAST			
SNACK			
LUNCH			
SNACK			
DINNER			

NOTES:

_____

_____

_____

_____

MY DAILY
CIDP

TODAY IS _____

WOKE UP FEELING
☺ ☺ ☺ ☺ ☺

I SLEPT (HOURS)
_____

I WOKE UP AT
_____

GOING TO BED FEELING
☺ ☺ ☺ ☺ ☺

I WAS ACTIVE (HOURS)
_____

I AM GOING TO BED AT
_____

TODAY I WOULD LIKE TO

01 _____

02 _____

03 _____

GOAL ACCOMPLISHED?

SYMPTOMS THIS MORNING

_____

_____

_____

_____

_____

_____

_____

_____

_____

SYMPTOMS THIS EVENING

_____

_____

_____

_____

_____

_____

_____

_____

_____

WATER ⬤⬤⬤⬤⬤⬤⬤⬤⬤   MEALS 🍽 🍽 🍽 🍽 🍽

BEFORE WORKOUT

AFTER WORKOUT

TARGET WORKOUT LENGTH: _____

ACTUAL WORKOUT LENGTH: _____

EXERCISE	SETS	REPS	RESISTANCE AMOUNT & TYPE

MEAL		PORTION	TIME
BREAKFAST			
SNACK			
LUNCH			
SNACK			
DINNER			

NOTES:

_____

_____

_____

_____

MY DAILY
CIDP

TODAY IS _____

WOKE UP FEELING

☺ ☺ ☺ ☹ ☹

I SLEPT (HOURS)
_____

I WOKE UP AT
_____

GOING TO BED FEELING

☺ ☺ ☺ ☹ ☹

I WAS ACTIVE (HOURS)
_____

I AM GOING TO BED AT
_____

TODAY I WOULD LIKE TO

GOAL ACCOMPLISHED?

01 _____

02 _____

03 _____

SYMPTOMS THIS MORNING

_____
_____
_____
_____
_____
_____
_____
_____
_____

SYMPTOMS THIS EVENING

_____
_____
_____
_____
_____
_____
_____
_____
_____

WATER ○○○○○○○○○   MEALS 🍽️🍽️🍽️🍽️🍽️

MY DAILY
CIDP

BEFORE WORKOUT

AFTER WORKOUT

TARGET WORKOUT LENGTH: _____

ACTUAL WORKOUT LENGTH: _____

EXERCISE	SETS	REPS	RESISTANCE AMOUNT & TYPE

MEAL		PORTION	TIME
BREAKFAST			
SNACK			
LUNCH			
SNACK			
DINNER			

NOTES:

_____

_____

_____

_____

MY DAILY
CIDP

TODAY IS _____

WOKE UP FEELING

☺ ☺ ☺ ☹ ☹

I SLEPT (HOURS)
_____

I WOKE UP AT
_____

GOING TO BED FEELING

☺ ☺ ☺ ☹ ☹

I WAS ACTIVE (HOURS)
_____

I AM GOING TO BED AT
_____

TODAY I WOULD LIKE TO   **GOAL ACCOMPLISHED?**

01 _____

02 _____

03 _____

SYMPTOMS THIS MORNING   **SYMPTOMS THIS EVENING**

_____   _____

_____   _____

_____   _____

_____   _____

_____   _____

_____   _____

_____   _____

_____   _____

_____   _____

WATER ⬡⬡⬡⬡⬡⬡⬡⬡   MEALS 🍴🍴🍴🍴🍴

MY DAILY
CIDP

BEFORE WORKOUT

TARGET WORKOUT LENGTH: _____

AFTER WORKOUT

ACTUAL WORKOUT LENGTH: _____

EXERCISE	SETS	REPS	RESISTANCE AMOUNT & TYPE

MEAL		PORTION	TIME
BREAKFAST			
SNACK			
LUNCH			
SNACK			
DINNER			

NOTES:

_____

_____

_____

_____

MY DAILY
CIDP

TODAY IS _____

WOKE UP FEELING

☺ 🙂 😐 😣 😢

I SLEPT (HOURS)
_____

I WOKE UP AT
_____

GOING TO BED FEELING

☺ 🙂 😐 😣 😢

I WAS ACTIVE (HOURS)
_____

I AM GOING TO BED AT
_____

TODAY I WOULD LIKE TO

GOAL ACCOMPLISHED?

01 _____

02 _____

03 _____

SYMPTOMS THIS MORNING

_____
_____
_____
_____
_____
_____
_____
_____
_____

SYMPTOMS THIS EVENING

_____
_____
_____
_____
_____
_____
_____
_____
_____

WATER ○○○○○○○○○

MEALS 🍽 🍽 🍽 🍽 🍽

MY DAILY
CIDP

BEFORE WORKOUT

AFTER WORKOUT

TARGET WORKOUT LENGTH: _____

ACTUAL WORKOUT LENGTH: _____

EXERCISE	SETS	REPS	RESISTANCE AMOUNT & TYPE

MEAL		PORTION	TIME
BREAKFAST			
SNACK			
LUNCH			
SNACK			
DINNER			

NOTES:

_____

_____

_____

_____

CIDP

TODAY IS _____

WOKE UP FEELING

☺ ☹ 😐 😠 😢

I SLEPT (HOURS) _____

I WOKE UP AT _____

GOING TO BED FEELING

☺ ☹ 😐 😠 😢

I WAS ACTIVE (HOURS) _____

I AM GOING TO BED AT _____

TODAY I WOULD LIKE TO

GOAL ACCOMPLISHED?

01 _____

02 _____

03 _____

SYMPTOMS THIS MORNING

_____
_____
_____
_____
_____
_____
_____
_____
_____

SYMPTOMS THIS EVENING

_____
_____
_____
_____
_____
_____
_____
_____
_____

WATER ⬦⬦⬦⬦⬦⬦⬦⬦⬦   MEALS 🍽🍽🍽🍽🍽

MY DAILY
CIDP

BEFORE WORKOUT

AFTER WORKOUT

TARGET WORKOUT LENGTH: _____

ACTUAL WORKOUT LENGTH: _____

EXERCISE	SETS	REPS	RESISTANCE AMOUNT & TYPE

MEAL		PORTION	TIME
BREAKFAST			
SNACK			
LUNCH			
SNACK			
DINNER			

NOTES:

_____

_____

_____

_____

MY DAILY
CIDP

TODAY IS _____

WOKE UP FEELING

☺ ☺ ☺ ☺ ☺

I SLEPT (HOURS)
_____

I WOKE UP AT
_____

GOING TO BED FEELING

☺ ☺ ☺ ☺ ☺

I WAS ACTIVE (HOURS)
_____

I AM GOING TO BED AT
_____

TODAY I WOULD LIKE TO   GOAL ACCOMPLISHED?

01 _____

02 _____

03 _____

SYMPTOMS THIS MORNING

_____
_____
_____
_____
_____
_____
_____
_____
_____

SYMPTOMS THIS EVENING

_____
_____
_____
_____
_____
_____
_____
_____
_____

WATER ◊ ◊ ◊ ◊ ◊ ◊ ◊ ◊   MEALS 🍽 🍽 🍽 🍽 🍽

MY DAILY
CIDP

BEFORE WORKOUT

TARGET WORKOUT LENGTH: _____

AFTER WORKOUT

ACTUAL WORKOUT LENGTH: _____

EXERCISE	SETS	REPS	RESISTANCE AMOUNT & TYPE

MEAL		PORTION	TIME
BREAKFAST			
SNACK			
LUNCH			
SNACK			
DINNER			

NOTES:

_____

_____

_____

_____

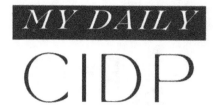

MY DAILY
CIDP

TODAY IS _____

WOKE UP FEELING	GOING TO BED FEELING
😃 🙂 😐 😠 😢	😃 🙂 😐 😠 😢

I SLEPT (HOURS)
_____

I WOKE UP AT
_____

I WAS ACTIVE (HOURS)
_____

I AM GOING TO BED AT
_____

TODAY I WOULD LIKE TO   GOAL ACCOMPLISHED?
_____

01
_____

02
_____

03
_____

SYMPTOMS THIS MORNING	SYMPTOMS THIS EVENING
_____	_____
_____	_____
_____	_____
_____	_____
_____	_____
_____	_____
_____	_____
_____	_____
_____	_____

WATER ○○○○○○○○○   MEALS 🍽 🍽 🍽 🍽 🍽

MY DAILY

CIDP

BEFORE WORKOUT

TARGET WORKOUT LENGTH: _____

AFTER WORKOUT

ACTUAL WORKOUT LENGTH: _____

EXERCISE	SETS	REPS	RESISTANCE AMOUNT & TYPE

MEAL		PORTION	TIME
BREAKFAST			
SNACK			
LUNCH			
SNACK			
DINNER			

NOTES:

_____

_____

_____

_____

CIDP

TODAY IS _____

WOKE UP FEELING

☺ ☺ ☺ ☹ ☹

I SLEPT (HOURS) _____

I WOKE UP AT _____

GOING TO BED FEELING

☺ ☺ ☺ ☹ ☹

I WAS ACTIVE (HOURS) _____

I AM GOING TO BED AT _____

TODAY I WOULD LIKE TO

GOAL ACCOMPLISHED?

01 _____

02 _____

03 _____

SYMPTOMS THIS MORNING

_____

_____

_____

_____

_____

_____

_____

_____

SYMPTOMS THIS EVENING

_____

_____

_____

_____

_____

_____

_____

_____

WATER ◊◊◊◊◊◊◊◊

MEALS 🍽 🍽 🍽 🍽 🍽

MY DAILY
CIDP

BEFORE WORKOUT

TARGET WORKOUT LENGTH: _____

AFTER WORKOUT

ACTUAL WORKOUT LENGTH: _____

EXERCISE	SETS	REPS	RESISTANCE AMOUNT & TYPE

MEAL		PORTION	TIME
BREAKFAST			
SNACK			
LUNCH			
SNACK			
DINNER			

NOTES:

_____

_____

_____

_____

CIDP

TODAY IS _____

WOKE UP FEELING

☺ ☹ 😐 😠 😢

I SLEPT (HOURS)
_____

I WOKE UP AT
_____

GOING TO BED FEELING

☺ ☹ 😐 😠 😢

I WAS ACTIVE (HOURS)
_____

I AM GOING TO BED AT
_____

TODAY I WOULD LIKE TO

GOAL ACCOMPLISHED?

01 _____

02 _____

03 _____

SYMPTOMS THIS MORNING

_____
_____
_____
_____
_____
_____
_____
_____
_____

SYMPTOMS THIS EVENING

_____
_____
_____
_____
_____
_____
_____
_____
_____

WATER ◊ ◊ ◊ ◊ ◊ ◊ ◊ ◊

MEALS 🍽 🍽 🍽 🍽 🍽

MY DAILY

CIDP

BEFORE WORKOUT

TARGET WORKOUT LENGTH: _____

AFTER WORKOUT

ACTUAL WORKOUT LENGTH: _____

EXERCISE	SETS	REPS	RESISTANCE AMOUNT & TYPE

MEAL		PORTION	TIME
BREAKFAST			
SNACK			
LUNCH			
SNACK			
DINNER			

NOTES:

_____

_____

_____

_____

MY DAILY
CIDP

TODAY IS _____

WOKE UP FEELING

☺ 🙂 😐 😠 😢

I SLEPT (HOURS) _____

I WOKE UP AT _____

GOING TO BED FEELING

☺ 🙂 😐 😠 😢

I WAS ACTIVE (HOURS) _____

I AM GOING TO BED AT _____

TODAY I WOULD LIKE TO

GOAL ACCOMPLISHED?

01 _____

02 _____

03 _____

SYMPTOMS THIS MORNING

_____
_____
_____
_____
_____
_____
_____
_____

SYMPTOMS THIS EVENING

_____
_____
_____
_____
_____
_____
_____
_____

WATER ◇◇◇◇◇◇◇◇◇   MEALS 🍽🍽🍽🍽🍽

CIDP

BEFORE WORKOUT

AFTER WORKOUT

TARGET WORKOUT LENGTH: _____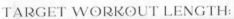

ACTUAL WORKOUT LENGTH: _____

EXERCISE	SETS	REPS	RESISTANCE AMOUNT & TYPE

MEAL		PORTION	TIME
BREAKFAST			
SNACK			
LUNCH			
SNACK			
DINNER			

NOTES:

_____

_____

_____

_____

MY DAILY
CIDP

TODAY IS _____

WOKE UP FEELING

☺ ☹ 😐 😠 😢

I SLEPT (HOURS)
_____

I WOKE UP AT
_____

GOING TO BED FEELING

☺ ☹ 😐 😠 😢

I WAS ACTIVE (HOURS)
_____

I AM GOING TO BED AT
_____

TODAY I WOULD LIKE TO

GOAL ACCOMPLISHED?

01 _____

02 _____

03 _____

SYMPTOMS THIS MORNING

_____
_____
_____
_____
_____
_____
_____
_____

SYMPTOMS THIS EVENING

_____
_____
_____
_____
_____
_____
_____
_____

WATER ○○○○○○○○○   MEALS 🍽 🍽 🍽 🍽 🍽

MY DAILY
CIDP

BEFORE WORKOUT

AFTER WORKOUT

TARGET WORKOUT LENGTH: _____

ACTUAL WORKOUT LENGTH: _____

EXERCISE	SETS	REPS	RESISTANCE AMOUNT & TYPE

MEAL		PORTION	TIME
BREAKFAST			
SNACK			
LUNCH			
SNACK			
DINNER			

NOTES:

_____

_____

_____

_____

CIDP

TODAY IS _____

WOKE UP FEELING

☺ ☺ ☺ ☹ ☹

I SLEPT (HOURS)
_____

I WOKE UP AT
_____

GOING TO BED FEELING

☺ ☺ ☺ ☹ ☹

I WAS ACTIVE (HOURS)
_____

I AM GOING TO BED AT
_____

TODAY I WOULD LIKE TO

GOAL ACCOMPLISHED?

01 _____

02 _____

03 _____

SYMPTOMS THIS MORNING

_____
_____
_____
_____
_____
_____
_____
_____
_____

SYMPTOMS THIS EVENING

_____
_____
_____
_____
_____
_____
_____
_____
_____

WATER ○○○○○○○○○

MEALS 🍽 🍽 🍽 🍽 🍽

MY DAILY
CIDP

BEFORE WORKOUT

AFTER WORKOUT

TARGET WORKOUT LENGTH: _____   ACTUAL WORKOUT LENGTH: _____

EXERCISE	SETS	REPS	RESISTANCE AMOUNT & TYPE

MEAL		PORTION	TIME
BREAKFAST			
SNACK			
LUNCH			
SNACK			
DINNER			

NOTES:

_____

_____

_____

_____

MY DAILY
CIDP

TODAY IS _____

WOKE UP FEELING
☺ ☹ 😐 😠 😢

GOING TO BED FEELING
☺ ☹ 😐 😠 😢

I SLEPT (HOURS)
_____

I WAS ACTIVE (HOURS)
_____

I WOKE UP AT
_____

I AM GOING TO BED AT
_____

TODAY I WOULD LIKE TO

GOAL ACCOMPLISHED?

01 _____

02 _____

03 _____

SYMPTOMS THIS MORNING

_____
_____
_____
_____
_____
_____
_____
_____

SYMPTOMS THIS EVENING

_____
_____
_____
_____
_____
_____
_____
_____

WATER ○○○○○○○○○

MEALS 🍽 🍽 🍽 🍽 🍽

MY DAILY
CIDP

BEFORE WORKOUT

AFTER WORKOUT

TARGET WORKOUT LENGTH: _____

ACTUAL WORKOUT LENGTH: _____

EXERCISE	SETS	REPS	RESISTANCE AMOUNT & TYPE

MEAL		PORTION	TIME
BREAKFAST			
SNACK			
LUNCH			
SNACK			
DINNER			

NOTES:

_____

_____

_____

_____

MY DAILY
CIDP

TODAY IS _____

WOKE UP FEELING

☺ ☺ ☺ ☺ ☺

I SLEPT (HOURS) _____

I WOKE UP AT _____

GOING TO BED FEELING

☺ ☺ ☺ ☺ ☺

I WAS ACTIVE (HOURS) _____

I AM GOING TO BED AT _____

TODAY I WOULD LIKE TO

GOAL ACCOMPLISHED?

01 _____

02 _____

03 _____

SYMPTOMS THIS MORNING

_____

_____

_____

_____

_____

_____

_____

_____

_____

SYMPTOMS THIS EVENING

_____

_____

_____

_____

_____

_____

_____

_____

_____

WATER ○○○○○○○○○   MEALS 🍽 🍽 🍽 🍽 🍽

MY DAILY
CIDP

BEFORE WORKOUT

AFTER WORKOUT

TARGET WORKOUT LENGTH: _____

ACTUAL WORKOUT LENGTH: _____

EXERCISE	SETS	REPS	RESISTANCE AMOUNT & TYPE

MEAL		PORTION	TIME
BREAKFAST			
SNACK			
LUNCH			
SNACK			
DINNER			

NOTES:

_____

_____

_____

_____

TODAY IS _____

WOKE UP FEELING

☺ ☹ ☺ ☹ ☹

I SLEPT (HOURS)
_____

I WOKE UP AT
_____

GOING TO BED FEELING

☺ ☹ ☺ ☹ ☹

I WAS ACTIVE (HOURS)
_____

I AM GOING TO BED AT
_____

TODAY I WOULD LIKE TO   GOAL ACCOMPLISHED?

01 _____

02 _____

03 _____

SYMPTOMS THIS MORNING

_____

_____

_____

_____

_____

_____

_____

_____

_____

SYMPTOMS THIS EVENING

_____

_____

_____

_____

_____

_____

_____

_____

_____

WATER ○○○○○○○○○   MEALS 🍽 🍽 🍽 🍽 🍽

MY DAILY
CIDP

BEFORE WORKOUT

AFTER WORKOUT

TARGET WORKOUT LENGTH: _____

ACTUAL WORKOUT LENGTH: _____

EXERCISE	SETS	REPS	RESISTANCE AMOUNT & TYPE

MEAL		PORTION	TIME
BREAKFAST			
SNACK			
LUNCH			
SNACK			
DINNER			

NOTES:

_____

_____

_____

_____

CIDP

TODAY IS _____

WOKE UP FEELING

☺ 🙂 😐 😠 😢

I SLEPT (HOURS)
_____

I WOKE UP AT
_____

GOING TO BED FEELING

☺ 🙂 😐 😠 😢

I WAS ACTIVE (HOURS)
_____

I AM GOING TO BED AT
_____

TODAY I WOULD LIKE TO   **GOAL ACCOMPLISHED?**
_____

01 _____

02 _____

03 _____

SYMPTOMS THIS MORNING   **SYMPTOMS THIS EVENING**

_____   _____

_____   _____

_____   _____

_____   _____

_____   _____

_____   _____

_____   _____

_____   _____

WATER ○○○○○○○○○   MEALS 🍽 🍽 🍽 🍽 🍽

MY DAILY
CIDP

BEFORE WORKOUT

TARGET WORKOUT LENGTH: _____

AFTER WORKOUT

ACTUAL WORKOUT LENGTH: _____

EXERCISE	SETS	REPS	RESISTANCE AMOUNT & TYPE

MEAL		PORTION	TIME
BREAKFAST			
SNACK			
LUNCH			
SNACK			
DINNER			

NOTES:

_____

_____

_____

MY DAILY
CIDP

TODAY IS _____

WOKE UP FEELING

☺ ☺ ☺ ☹ ☹

I SLEPT (HOURS)
_____

I WOKE UP AT
_____

GOING TO BED FEELING

☺ ☺ ☺ ☹ ☹

I WAS ACTIVE (HOURS)
_____

I AM GOING TO BED AT
_____

TODAY I WOULD LIKE TO

01 _____

02 _____

03 _____

GOAL ACCOMPLISHED?

_____

_____

_____

_____

SYMPTOMS THIS MORNING

_____

_____

_____

_____

_____

_____

_____

_____

SYMPTOMS THIS EVENING

_____

_____

_____

_____

_____

_____

_____

_____

WATER ○○○○○○○○○ MEALS 🍽 🍽 🍽 🍽 🍽

MY DAILY
CIDP

BEFORE WORKOUT

AFTER WORKOUT

TARGET WORKOUT LENGTH: _____

ACTUAL WORKOUT LENGTH: _____

EXERCISE	SETS	REPS	RESISTANCE AMOUNT & TYPE

MEAL		PORTION	TIME
BREAKFAST			
SNACK			
LUNCH			
SNACK			
DINNER			

NOTES:

_____

_____

_____

_____

MY DAILY
CIDP

TODAY IS _____

WOKE UP FEELING

☺ ☺ ☺ ☹ ☹

I SLEPT (HOURS)
_____

I WOKE UP AT
_____

GOING TO BED FEELING

☺ ☺ ☺ ☹ ☹

I WAS ACTIVE (HOURS)
_____

I AM GOING TO BED AT
_____

TODAY I WOULD LIKE TO   **GOAL ACCOMPLISHED?**

01 _____

02 _____

03 _____

SYMPTOMS THIS MORNING   **SYMPTOMS THIS EVENING**

_____   _____

_____   _____

_____   _____

_____   _____

_____   _____

_____   _____

_____   _____

_____   _____

WATER ⬭⬭⬭⬭⬭⬭⬭⬭   MEALS 🍽🍽🍽🍽🍽

MY DAILY
CIDP

BEFORE WORKOUT

TARGET WORKOUT LENGTH: _____

AFTER WORKOUT

ACTUAL WORKOUT LENGTH: _____

EXERCISE	SETS	REPS	RESISTANCE AMOUNT & TYPE

MEAL		PORTION	TIME
BREAKFAST			
SNACK			
LUNCH			
SNACK			
DINNER			

NOTES:

_____

_____

_____

_____

MY DAILY
CIDP

TODAY IS _____

WOKE UP FEELING

☺ ☺ ☺ ☹ ☹

I SLEPT (HOURS)
_____

I WOKE UP AT
_____

GOING TO BED FEELING

☺ ☺ ☺ ☹ ☹

I WAS ACTIVE (HOURS)
_____

I AM GOING TO BED AT
_____

TODAY I WOULD LIKE TO

GOAL ACCOMPLISHED?

01 _____

02 _____

03 _____

SYMPTOMS THIS MORNING

_____
_____
_____
_____
_____
_____
_____
_____

SYMPTOMS THIS EVENING

_____
_____
_____
_____
_____
_____
_____
_____

WATER ◇◇◇◇◇◇◇◇◇

MEALS 🍽 🍽 🍽 🍽 🍽

MY DAILY
CIDP

BEFORE WORKOUT

TARGET WORKOUT LENGTH: _____

AFTER WORKOUT

ACTUAL WORKOUT LENGTH: _____

EXERCISE	SETS	REPS	RESISTANCE AMOUNT & TYPE

MEAL		PORTION	TIME
BREAKFAST			
SNACK			
LUNCH			
SNACK			
DINNER			

NOTES:

_____

_____

_____

_____

MY DAILY
CIDP

TODAY IS _____

WOKE UP FEELING

☺ ☺ ☺ ☹ ☹

I SLEPT (HOURS)
_____

I WOKE UP AT
_____

GOING TO BED FEELING

☺ ☺ ☺ ☹ ☹

I WAS ACTIVE (HOURS)
_____

I AM GOING TO BED AT
_____

TODAY I WOULD LIKE TO

GOAL ACCOMPLISHED?

01 _____

02 _____

03 _____

SYMPTOMS THIS MORNING

_____

_____

_____

_____

_____

_____

_____

_____

_____

SYMPTOMS THIS EVENING

_____

_____

_____

_____

_____

_____

_____

_____

_____

WATER ◊◊◊◊◊◊◊◊◊

MEALS 🍴🍴🍴🍴🍴

MY DAILY
CIDP

BEFORE WORKOUT

AFTER WORKOUT

TARGET WORKOUT LENGTH: _____

ACTUAL WORKOUT LENGTH: _____

EXERCISE	SETS	REPS	RESISTANCE AMOUNT & TYPE

MEAL		PORTION	TIME
BREAKFAST			
SNACK			
LUNCH			
SNACK			
DINNER			

NOTES:

_____

_____

_____

_____

MY DAILY
CIDP

TODAY IS _____

WOKE UP FEELING
☺ ☺ ☺ ☹ ☹

I SLEPT (HOURS) _____

I WOKE UP AT _____

GOING TO BED FEELING
☺ ☺ ☺ ☹ ☹

I WAS ACTIVE (HOURS) _____

I AM GOING TO BED AT _____

TODAY I WOULD LIKE TO

01 _____

02 _____

03 _____

GOAL ACCOMPLISHED?

SYMPTOMS THIS MORNING

_____
_____
_____
_____
_____
_____
_____
_____

SYMPTOMS THIS EVENING

_____
_____
_____
_____
_____
_____
_____
_____

WATER ○○○○○○○○○ MEALS 🍽 🍽 🍽 🍽 🍽

MY DAILY
CIDP

BEFORE WORKOUT

TARGET WORKOUT LENGTH: _____

AFTER WORKOUT

ACTUAL WORKOUT LENGTH: _____

EXERCISE	SETS	REPS	RESISTANCE AMOUNT & TYPE

MEAL		PORTION	TIME
BREAKFAST			
SNACK			
LUNCH			
SNACK			
DINNER			

NOTES:

_____

_____

_____

_____

MY DAILY
CIDP

WHAT I AM MOST PROUD OF

MY TOP ACHIEVEMENTS

FITNESS	NUTRITION	MIND

WHAT I WANT TO ACCOMPLISH NEXT

MY DAILY

CIDP

NOTES

CIDP

NOTES

Printed in the USA
CPSIA information can be obtained
at www.ICGtesting.com
LVHW010210131023
760673LV00062B/1258

9 781088 153949